Abandoned Pregnant
A Self-Help Guide For Women Going Through Pregnancy Alone

KANDY DOLOR

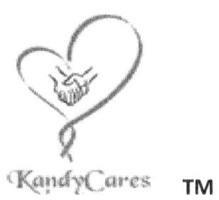

TM

Abandoned Pregnant

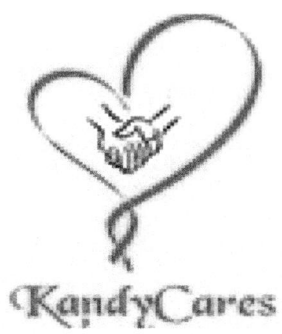

Abandoned Pregnant

First published in Great Britain by KandyCares
Copyright©2015 by Kandy Dolor

All rights reserved. No part of this publication may be reproduced, distributed, or transmitted in any form or by any means, including photocopying, recording, or other electronic or mechanical methods, without the prior written permission of the publisher, except in the case of brief quotations embodied in critical reviews and certain other noncommercial uses permitted by copyright law.

www.kandycares.org
www.facebook.com/KandyCaresSelfHelpBooks

A catalogue record for this book is available from the British Library.

ISBN:978-0-9934787-0-3

Abandoned Pregnant

Acknowledgments

I dedicate this book to women who have gone through pregnancy alone.

To my mum,
Thank you for inspiring and pushing me. I love you.

To Ava Brown,
Thank you for all of your continuous support and for editing my book free of charge, I am forever grateful.

Abandoned Pregnant

To Savannah & Dayren,

Bringing you both into the world was two of the best choices I ever made in my life.
I love you both very much.
Even when you are adults, you will both always be my babies.

Abandoned Pregnant

Preface

I began writing this book during my first pregnancy but stopped, because I felt overwhelmed by anger and didn't want to continue.

The second time around, when I found myself yet again pregnant and abandoned, I had so much to say about it that I knew I had to carry on writing.

I can remember sitting on the floor of my living room, eight months pregnant, in tears and in incomplete disbelief over how my life had come to this. I failed to understand, how could the man – who, I believed, once loved and cared about me – just up and leave me because I was pregnant? Furthermore, how could he not be interested in his own baby?
I experienced unwanted thoughts and feelings, such as anger and the need for revenge. There would be a few days in the week when I missed my ex and wanted him back; the other few days, I would feel nothing but hatred towards him and could have happily lived my life without ever seeing him again.
Sometimes when I thought about my situation and became hyper, I'd start calling or texting him, only to end up feeling rejected and hot-headed. Usually, he would ignore me; as if I didn't even exist in his life anymore.

Abandoned Pregnant

Whenever he denied to engage in any communication with me he was cold, disrespectful and plain nasty; I would always feel a lot worse than I had done before I got in touch with him.

I will never forget the day I uploaded a hugely embarrassing picture of my ex on my Blackberry Messenger profile picture: I displayed it for all my contacts to see - including him.
I really wanted him to experience some of the frustration that I was dealing with.
I went through a whirlwind of emotions that I knew weren't good for me, but I just couldn't control it, or help myself.
Deep down, I used to wish my ex would come back to me so that we could become a family.
Looking back on it, I know I was such a silly girl; my ex didn't care about the affects his actions had on me and he wasn't getting himself into disarray like I was... in fact, he was out there seeing other women and very thing I was doing was just pushing him further away from me.
I had to get strong and pull myself together pretty quickly, which meant having to let go of my ex, what he had done to me and holding myself accountable for my own actions also.

I got ready for my baby's arrival and focused on what was important, it was not without great effort, but I did it – twice.

Abandoned Pregnant

You can do it too.

I wrote this book to help women facing similar situations to the one I've been through.
I have written a combination of my experiences and my struggles during both my pregnancies. I have included advice on how to cope with many things that may arise when you find yourself in a dilemma such as this.
I have also given insight into how I managed.
I hope readers take some sort of comfort from my self-help book.

Know that you are not alone, how you feel now will not last forever; you will get through this and guess what? You'll be a stronger woman because of it.

Abandoned Pregnant

Chapter 1 – P10
Single & Pregnant

Chapter 2 – P20
Why Me

Chapter 3 –P30
Wishing He Would Come Back

Chapter 4 –P36
He's Moved On

Chapter 5 –P44
Coping With Rejection

Chapter 6 –P50
Give Up Trying To Make Your Ex See Sense

Chapter 7 –P56
Revenge

Chapter 8 –P62
When Will I Stop Feeling This Way

Chapter 9 –P67
Accepting Things As They Are

Abandoned Pregnant

Chapter 10 –P73
Learning From This Experience

Chapter 11 –P78
Letting Go

Chapter 12 -P88
Love Yourself

Chapter 13 –P93
Moving On

Chapter 14 –P97
What Do You Tell Your Child About Daddy

Chapter 15 –P104
New Relationships

Chapter 16 –P104
Contact With His Family

Chapter 17 –P111
Sudden Contact With Your Ex

Chapter 18 –P118
Reconciling With Your Ex

Chapter 19 –P123
Be Grateful For What You do Have

Abandoned Pregnant

Chapter 20 -P126
Coping With Depression

Chapter 21- P132
You Will Survive

Chapter 1
Pregnant & Single

No woman wants to be abandoned by her partner at any time, let alone during a pregnancy. And the very last thing we desire is for our child to be brought up without a father.
I am sure you imagined as a little girl –I like most women have – that you would be married before having children, or that your partner would gaze at you, looking delighted when you broke the news about your pregnancy to him. You probably imagined every romantic scenario; anything except him doing a runner from his own baby, behaving like a complete coward, and leaving you to go through it all alone.
Everyone knows that accidents do happen and not all pregnancies are planned, but some take it well, some don't.
When a man is totally turning his back on you, he could have many reasons.

He might have wanted you to end a pregnancy and you have decided to go ahead with.
If this is the case – if your ex wanted you to have an abortion - and you have made the decision to keep your baby? High five, that's amazing.

Abandoned Pregnant

Once you choose to have an abortion you can't go back, and you have to live with it if it's not what you really wanted deep down.
Bear that in mind: terminating a pregnancy for a partner will not save a relationship. Everything won't just go back to normal: it leads to resentment, distress, potential depression and a loss of mistrust.

Another reason could be that the two of you weren't in a committed relationship. If what you had with this man was causal - and assuming the pregnancy was unexpected - then you should expect nothing from this guy. He could take you by surprise, but life isn't a fairy tale.
Unfortunately, you both took a gamble when you entered into casual sex - for however long that might have been for - and you will now have to deal with your actions, taking into account the best thing for your baby.

Your ex could say that he doesn't want to have a baby, or he could also be horribly cruel in letting you know that he doesn't want to have a baby with *you,* specifically.
If he really did not want to have a child he should have insisted on using contraception all the time; they don't always work though.

Abandoned Pregnant

Anyway, whatever his reasons, no matter how pathetic they may sound, the most important thing at this very moment is that you have a *life* inside you.
You have to forget about him. You don't need anything from him, he might be wanted, but he is not needed.
Now is the time for change, the biggest adjustment of your life is fast approaching just months away.

I understand your pain.
Your baby is not coming into the best situation, you more than likely have wished all sorts of bad karma on your ex and called him every name in the book.
The whole situation just feels like such a mess in your head whenever you think about it...

Don't suppress your emotions, if you want to cry, then cry; if you want to burn every single picture you have of him, go ahead!
Right now your emotions are all over the place, it's a part of being pregnant, and it won't last.
In the beginning, you should allow yourself to 'feel it' and take each day as it comes, while gradually trying to take control of your emotions. Yes, what he is doing is wrong, but you are not in control of that; however, you are in control of how you react to it.
Although men do think differently than women, a man definitely understands what he's doing when he rejects a woman who is carrying his child.
He knows that his actions are wrong.

Abandoned Pregnant

The horrible truth of it is, if he chooses to do so anyway, he doesn't care.
He does not care about you, your pregnancy or the baby.
He only cares about himself.
However, your ex is still only human, he does have feelings too and a conscience; the guilt will catch up with him in one way or another, even if you never find out about it.
You can never get back in time, regret is not a very good thing to live with at all and you never know what the future holds so don't judge today's situation as the norm for the rest of your life. Know that a reluctant father can change his mind.
Your ex could reconsider his involvement at any time, and if you think you are likely to allow him to have contact with your baby or to end up getting back together with him, then I want you to think seriously about all the stress and anxiety that you are putting on yourself and your unborn baby over him at this very moment.
Will it all be worth it in a few months, or a year?

However, do not put your hopes on him wanting to make up, as there is a good chance that it won't happen. No one in their right mind would risk losing someone they love forever if they wanted to keep that person in their life.
Don't wait for him to come back: This guy has proven that you cannot place any expectations on him, and

doing so regardless is what will end up breaking your heart, over and over.

The only thing you can do is be strong, for yourself and for your baby, figure out how you will provide for your child alone.

A positive attitude is a must.

It is also important that you enjoy your time being pregnant; don't spend it being miserable.

Even if you were with your ex right now, you would still be going through all the hormonal and physical changes alone; that is because this pregnancy is yours, so OWN it, it's your experience.

Notice all the wonderful changes that are happening inside of you and spend some time relaxing by yourself!

You will never be alone again in a few months.

Paint your toe nails before your tummy is too big for you to be able to do it yourself, watch catch-ups or old re-runs of your favourite soaps, movies or TV series, google interesting facts and things, read about what your baby is doing and how he or she is growing and developing inside of you.

Treat yourself to a pregnancy massage; if you want something a little less costly purchase a foot massager or some Mum To Be pamper products.

Do not stop cooking for yourself just because your ex isn't around anymore! You are eating for two now and take-out on a regular basis cannot be an option anymore, not only is it unhealthy, but, you would also be putting your unborn baby at risk of food poisoning, so make sure you...

Abandoned Pregnant

<u>Eat healthy!</u>
Find out what kind of food is good for you during your pregnancy.
<u>Sleep!</u>
Take advantage of uninterrupted sleep.
Indulge in quality time with your duvet, for the days are coming when it will be all over.
<u>Do things that make you happy!</u>
Relax as much as you can because soon, you will be up changing nappies, making bottles, singing lullaby's and spending hours just gazing at your baby in absolute amazement.

Spend some time looking up online information about things you can do to keep busy – such as exercise classes, antenatal classes, pregnancy groups etc.
Attending antenatal classes and other groups doesn't mean that you have no idea of what you are doing: it just shows you want to become the best mum you can possibly be.
If you can find a support group to attend at one of your local community centres, you may even find other mothers who are in a similar situation and you may not feel so alone if you have someone to talk to who can relate to what you are going through. You would be surprised to discover how much strength and support you receive from other mums.
If you have friends you can talk to that is great, but friends don't always understand – unless it has

happened or is happening to them – and can make you feel like if you bring 'him' up again you haven't moved on; or that they have heard you talk about him so many times they now seem to appear bored and uninterested.

Family members are good to speak to when you are close enough and trust that you can share your feelings with them; if they have been generally supportive of you in the past then there is no reason why they should stop now, at a time when you need their help more than ever.

When it comes down to your delivery, you should think about who you would like to be there to support you, who you think is the best person for the job.

A good birthing partner can make all the difference during your labour, they should be there to provide encouragement and should also be confident enough to make sure all your needs are being met.

Most hospitals allow two people present, but don't agree to have anybody who you don't want there tagging along: say a nice, but firm no. The most important thing is that you are happy with your choice and feel comfortable.

After going through giving birth you may feel wrecked. Try to get as much rest as you can.

It takes time to recover from having a baby.

I'm not going to paint a rosy picture of being a single mum - as time passes, the 247 job does have its bad sides; not everyone will tell you about because they want you to believe that they are doing just fine.

Of course being a mother is a true blessing: your life is full of hugs and kisses, laughter, cute stuff, and so many more things that would have anybody saying 'Awwww!' But there are other parts to it.

If nobody speaks about the reality of single motherhood then women will go into it without knowing what is ahead of them.

The facts are: there will be days when you might feel exhausted from all the hard work, days when you may worry, days when the tasks of being a single mum are totally relentless.

If most women knew how much of a struggle it trying to look after a child is on a one salary they would think again about their choices.

Being a single mum is very hard at times, but it is doable.

Yes, it is tough and can be lonely, but it will also be the best thing you ever do in your life and the most rewarding thing in the world. Your children will love you for it in the end and all those sleepless nights will be worth it.

You may even find that as your child gets older, communication between you both is very open, thanks to that one to one family dynamic.

POWER TO ALL SINGLE MOTHERS!

Abandoned Pregnant

I was down and depressed for quite some time during my first pregnancy – due to my ex leaving me and not wanting to have anything to do with my pregnancy.
I couldn't stop thinking about him and it really hurt me badly; I could not believe he had done that to me.
All the times he said he loved me kept going round and round in my head; all the lovely things he had done for me... I had so much to show for our relationship and I didn't understand it at all. I spent a lot of wasted time trying to figure out his behaviour.
I put so much stress on myself and I drove myself crazy, wishing that he would come back to me and tell me he'd made a mistake; that he would just say how much he missed me, and how sorry he was.
I even went as far as to foolishly call several psychic lines to ask them if he would come back to me - which they said he would.

As time passed, it got easier.
I kept myself busy, read a lot and wrote loads; in fact it was then I first started this book.
I was often around members of his family and grew close to his mother: even though my ex didn't want to have any involvement with me, at that time his family did and they were totally supportive.

I attended antenatal classes during my pregnancy.
It was very good as I learned a lot

Abandoned Pregnant

(I'd recommend it especially if you don't know CPR) and it also made the fact I wasn't *just* pregnant but also going to have an actual baby so real! The whole thing suddenly hit me: I was going to be a mum.

In the early stages of my pregnancy I didn't attend any support groups in person, but I did get support through online forums and chat groups.
Not everyone was understanding though: some were an unsympathetic group of listeners making comments like "I made my bed and I had to lay in it."
The reason I turned to online support was because I was sure my friends had heard me talk about my situation too much and I was slowly becoming 'that friend with issues' so I learned to vent my frustration to strangers instead - obviously keeping my identity anonymous.
At the time, I was fuming with whoever those strangers were for not understanding the pain I was in, but after going through my second pregnancy alone it was then I finally understood what they meant.
Shame it took me a second time to learn from my mistakes but better late than never.

Chapter 2: Why Me?

Being pregnant with an ex's child is bound to be hard on any woman, especially if she still has feelings for the father.

You might cry yourself to sleep, you might feel down, there will be good days and bad days, but remember: you made the choice to keep your baby, don't regret your decision.
It is by far the easiest of predicaments to be in, but, in time, you will become used to your ex partner's absence and you will start to forget that your baby even has a father!
The fact is: you don't need a man who has deserted you while you were pregnant. If he could do this to you, it would be worse if he stayed.
I know there will be times when the only thing you can think of is your ex, you may wonder what he is doing and who he is seeing.
Do not do it to yourself: he will be in control. You will give him all the power by having him on your mind, along with all these questions that you cannot answer.
You may never get the answers, and even if you did,
I doubt they would make you feel any better.
The truth hurts.
There may be times when you might feel embarrassed being in the company of certain people who know

Abandoned Pregnant

about the situation you are in, but unless these people are providing a roof over your head, feeding or clothing you, or will be taking on board any responsibilities in helping you with your baby, then you owe them no explanation. You don't have to let them know; unless you choose to.

I understand how upsetting it is when you feel that others may be speaking about what is happening to you behind your back, or when you suspect some people might have lost their respect towards you and look down on you now that you are a single parent.

Sometimes you are judged for the choice you made in your partner.

It is not a nice feeling at all, but if anybody is speaking about you, that is their business, not yours.

I know it is frustrating, but do not allow gossip get to you.

Ever heard of the saying 'Today for me, Tomorrow for you?'

Suppose you are out shopping and you bump into an old friend who you haven't seen in ages.

She congratulates you on noticing your bump, she makes a nosy comment such as 'your other half must be so happy'

What do you say?

Nothing.

Simply smile and say something like 'oh yes, everyone is happy.'

Abandoned Pregnant

You do not need to explain what is really going on in your life.
Most of us know our neighbours, even if we just say hello and make the odd comment about the weather.
Some neighbours do indeed gossip and you may well be the talk of the street once you are showing and are noticeably pregnant while your ex is nowhere in sight.
These people are irrelevant. They play no part in your child's life, so do not pay any mind to their chatter if you get wind of it.
It never helps to defend yourself against cruel gossip so just let them talk and keep your head up.
Not everybody will be criticising you; I'm sure you will hear more expressions of praise and support than negative comments.
Some people really do care about what you are going through and will be sympathetic to your situation, they may understand what it is like and how hard it is; when you receive kind gestures and offers of help, don't be afraid to accept the help it if you need it.

When it comes down to announcing the news to family members, let's face it: it can be difficult. They are not likely to be very happy with the situation you are in, but hopefully they will be supportive of your decisions and will try to help you as much as they can.
Some individuals in your family may even try to talk you out of your pregnancy if you are not too far gone. Any decisions you make must be YOUR OWN, YOU have to live with the choices you make, not anybody else.

Abandoned Pregnant

If your ex has family members who are aware of your pregnancy and have expressed their wishes to be involved in your child's life then by all means let them if they are genuine and are going to be of any help.
At the end of the day, whatever the circumstance, remember: the decision is yours to make.

It's time to face some very extremely painful facts: your ex is more than likely to be seeing someone else by now, even if it's not anything serious.
If friends mention that they have seen him around and try to fill you in on what he has been up to, politely inform them that you do not want to hear about it. , If they hear any gossip involving him and you'd really prefer not to know anything, tell them that you would appreciate it if they kindly prevent themselves from sharing it, as you are not interested in anything he is doing.
Your priority is your child, he is none of your concern anymore.
Of course it is easier said than done, but like I mentioned before, it is about learning to control your emotions, your thoughts, and your feelings, they all belong to you. You are in charge.
If you do find yourself getting caught up thinking about him, and cannot seem to get a grasp on anything to distract yourself, try reading this book over to remind yourself of how much you really don't need him. Throw yourself into something new that's outside of your usual

comfort zone. The pain will get easier. Break ups are never easy, nor are they supposed to be.
This might sound harsh and you have most probably heard of this saying before 'You are not the first and you shall not be the last.'
Many women before you have been in the very same boat and they have survived; you will too, remember that.

Your baby could be a girl who will eventually grow up to become a woman; would you want your daughter wasting her emotions and her feelings on someone like your ex?
What advice would you give to her? How would you feel about it?
I am sure it would break your heart to know your daughter was being treated badly and there was nothing you could do about it, and I am certain you would be advising her to have nothing more to do with this man.
It is time to stop battling with yourself and accept what has happened: as painful as it is the sooner you face up to the reality of what you are dealing with, the sooner you can start to heal, and healing is important.
Speaking to a counsellor might be helpful to get all your feelings out; I strongly recommend going to see one, you can go through your doctor and ask to be referred.
Be very careful how you go about this though, as you do not want social services to be contacted unnecessarily.
Sad but true.

Abandoned Pregnant

With everything that is going on in the world, social services can never be too sure - now more than ever - and they have to follow up any concerns from doctors; it is protocol.
You can also search online for any organisations or charities offering free counselling in your area.
Relate Counselling also offer workshop activities.
Nowadays some organisations or private professionals offer counselling via Skype or over the phone, allowing you the advantage of speaking in the comfort of your own home. Most private counsellors offer a free consultation so you can get a 'feel' of if you think this is the right counsellor for you before you pay for any sessions.
Do your research before making any choices; and make sure you are speaking to a qualified counsellor.
You can also go to your local children's centre and enquire about seeing a counsellor.
All my advice given above is based on specifically UK residents.
If you live outside the UK you may have to go down other alternative routes to request counselling sessions.
Everything you are doing now, which should hopefully be maternity classes, a group for single pregnant mums, and counselling should all get you going in the right direction.
Not only will you be meeting new people and socialising with others who could also become potential friends, but you are also moving on.

Abandoned Pregnant

I've found some of my best friends at a maternity class and we've helped each other a number of times once our babies were here.
Even though things sometimes don't go the way we imagined, I believe that some of the bad things that happen to us really are blessings in disguise, and the rest are lessons to be learnt. What if that man had stayed with you? Knowing what you have now discovered about his character, I'm sure you realise that it wouldn't have been sunsets and rainbows.
I also believe that there is always a reason and a purpose for everything.
Life is not over because you are a pregnant single woman: one day, when the time is right, you will love again.
Until that day comes, put all your love, time and energy into raising your child and you won't go wrong.
It might seem a long way out of sight now, but time really does go so quickly; you can be happy again. It is down to you to believe it, though.
Make yourself content, better yourself: you are responsible for your own happiness.
We have one life and it is temporary, we don't know when our time is up, so it is important not to worry about the things that we can't change, or waste our time on people who don't care about us.
Unfortunately, your ex is one of those people and you need to accept it.
Holding on to someone you know for a fact does not care about you only holds you back in the end.

Abandoned Pregnant

You know your ex is no good for you. Let go.
It is the best thing you could ever do for yourself right now.

During the second trimester of my first pregnancy, I attended anger management and counselling sessions.
I felt so much hatred towards my ex, yet I still loved him and I was angry with myself for having those feelings, even though he was treating me so badly.
I felt like I was stupid and thought "no wonder I am in the situation I am in."
I didn't want to bring my baby into the world while harbouring all those negative feelings, and I decided that I should get help before my child came. A quick fix.
I was wrong. Do not go for counselling or anger management for a short time, as what you are going through has a long term effect on you, without you even realising it.
I cannot stress enough how important it is to let your feelings out and be heard: listen to yourself, and think 'wow I really went through all this' and you'll realise you will survive it.

I can recall standing at a bus stop one day and seeing a friend I'd lost touch with. She was also pregnant. When she asked me about my partner my first initial instinct was to be evasive, but something made me tell her the truth; maybe because of the closeness we once shared.

Abandoned Pregnant

It so happened that she also was in the same situation and after exchanging numbers, that night we spoke on the phone for hours. We met up regularly and it was sad to see my friend going through the same abandonment I felt but I admit it was nice to have someone to talk to, someone who genuinely understood. I would be there for her and she would be there for me.

My friend would call her ex way too much. Every minute, she was someone different: in one sentence she would tell him how much she missed him and in another, how much she hated him. Her behaviour slowly rubbed off onto me and I was calling my ex a lot more, trying to get him to speak to me, to no avail.

Eventually he changed his number. I went insane! I couldn't send him hate texts anymore or call him up and give him an earful while he remained silent. Even if I stopped shouting and said his name softly there would be silence, but then I would just text him. Now it was over, I couldn't contact him.

He must have gotten really fed up with me, thinking back on my behaviour now.

It was whilst speaking with my counsellor that I realised I had been causing myself even more pain and rejection by continuing to try to contact this man and it was by listening to my own words I realised how pathetically desperate I seemed. I had no dignity.

I had to keep myself distracted from thinking about him, so I stopped hanging around with my friend as she was only making matters worse.

Abandoned Pregnant

I went out, bought a few pregnancy books and started focusing on everything I needed for my baby's arrival. I also bought pampering products like relaxation soaks for the bath, creams, massage oils and a foot massager which really came in good use!

During my second pregnancy, whenever I couldn't stop thinking about my ex, I would distract myself by listening to relaxation music and positive affirmations. I'd also watch comedies that would have me laughing in no time.

I would Google different countries in the world and find out amazing and interesting facts about strange things that have no explanation.

I watched and read stuff that I wouldn't normally have tried and actually began to become interested in these things; whenever I was out I started to look forward to going home to either finish researching, reading something or writing. I no longer dreaded being alone, I was happy with my own company.

I didn't even notice I was becoming a different person, but I was.

Chapter 3
Wishing Your Ex Would Come Back

Some time may have passed since you last engaged in communication with your ex.
Your pregnancy is progressing further along and everything is starting to become more real.
As much as you may have tried to forget about him(and maybe for a while, you have) what you probably are struggling to get your head around right now is the fact he is still not back with you and that he might not be coming back, ever.
Maybe deep down inside you might have had some hope that he would have made contact by now, but every passing day is the same, regardless of how much time has gone by.
Stop waiting and wasting time.
Believe this is happening.
You are going to have a baby and you are going to do a great job at being a single parent; you don't need him.
Say it out loud 'I am going to do a great job at being a single parent, I don't need him'
Believe it.
I remember when I couldn't believe this was happening to me.

I was in denial for ages, secretly hoping my ex would show up unannounced one day, begging for my

forgiveness, praying he would see he had made a mistake.
I only made things worse for myself by not addressing the truth properly.
He was gone. He wasn't coming back and I just really couldn't believe it was happening to me.
I was left to be a single parent; to this very day and I am doing a great job at it. I don't need him and feel sick to my stomach when I think back to the times I used to beg my ex to be in his child's life.

Yes, there will be times where if you are having a bad day you will think of your child's father and become angry all over again, or start to wonder 'how can he not even care or want to know how I am doing, how my pregnancy is going?'
It is sad, but he does not care about you or his baby right now, the only person he cares about and is thinking of is himself.
And you could do well by taking a leaf out of his book by caring about yourself.
Remember that this is a point in your life where you have to make mature decisions, whether you feel mature or not.
It's time to plan ahead for your baby and for yourself not including him in the picture.
Make your surroundings stable.
This is also the time where you should get rid of anyone around you who you think is not genuine; cut them off, as well as anything else that's bad for you.

Abandoned Pregnant

You need to be around positivity.
We all get lonely, it can be a daunting feeling, especially when you are pregnant and full of hormones.
In your moment of loneliness it's inevitable that you will start to miss your ex, and it's horrible, you feel like you hate him but you love him too.
View your life as a puzzle that you are putting together, piece by piece to form a beautiful picture, your ex wasn't the right fit in your puzzle, so no matter how bad you want to squeeze him into the slot it isn't going to work.
Being pregnant, you deserve the support and companionship of the man who is the father of your child but deserving something doesn't mean that you'll get it.

I missed my ex so much in my first pregnancy, I would dream of him a lot.
In my second pregnancy, I was too angry to acknowledge that I did in fact miss my other ex, although I do remember one night I dreamt I was pulling him towards me to kiss him, only to wake up finding myself pulling at my poor daughter who was asleep next to me!
It is completely understandable if you do get lonely.
We all need love. Be patient.
Soon, you will have the greatest love of all in your arms: no other love can top or replace a mother's love for her child.

Abandoned Pregnant

Some women worry themselves silly by thinking that they will never find love again with a child, but that is not true. There are many broken families in the world – which is unfortunate, however, broken families can go on to create step-families.
There is no rush to meet someone new but when you do feel ready to do so, then you should have an idea of the type of man who is going to be good for you: his personality, values, qualities and what you would like to have in common that is important to you - don't settle for anybody who reminds of your ex!
Love yourself.
Don't ever think that you should be treated any less than you deserve just because you are a single parent.
At the first sign of anything that is wrong in a new relationship, don't stick around trying to change him or make things better.
Don't get yourself sucked into the whirlwind a second time round just because you feel lonely.
Leave immediately.

Being pregnant and alone for a second time with a child to look after - who you have to mask your sadness to in order to prevent them from knowing something is wrong - is hard, believe me.
When you feel lonely or vulnerable, pick up the phone and call a friend; make sure it's a supportive friend – who preferably doesn't have a partner that she would chat about, because that's the last thing you need!

Abandoned Pregnant

If a friend can come over to your house to keep you company, even better.
In case you don't feel like talking, watch a comedy that will get you laughing.
I read The Bible a lot when I was pregnant, especially when I felt sad and lonely; I can honestly say it lifted my spirits. I would always feel better after reading it, and it gave me hope.
I also would go onto a website where I could live chat, and volunteer to listen to young people's problems.
At the end of my conversations with the strangers, it reminded me that there were so many people in the world who are struggling with issues far worse than my own.
It was while I was reading these people's problems that I also remembered that there were so many women in the world who would give anything to be able to get pregnant and have a baby, and there I was with what these women wanted but I wasn't happy because I didn't have a man by my side.
There are some women who go for artificial insemination at sperm clinics; some choose not to know the identity of their baby's father and have no expectations from him therefore avoiding disappointment. They are prepared to raise their child alone and are happy to have the opportunity to be able to do so.
After I had thought of this, I was grateful and somewhat humbled.

Abandoned Pregnant

Try to remember how you once lived your life: before you met your ex, you were surviving just fine without him then, and you will survive just fine without him now too.
You will get over him and become stronger from it.
Letting go of a relationship is painful, however, it is not nearly as difficult as remaining in one whose time has passed.
Every relationship has a natural life span.
Some people only come into our lives to teach us lessons that we are meant to learn; they put us through situations or experiences that we are just supposed to have happen to us on our journey in life.
Not everyone who comes into your life will have a purpose to stay in it.
We can trust that in time a greater understanding will come to us, even though we may not understand the lesson today.

Chapter 4
He's Moved On

Finding out that your ex is in a new relationship can cause deep feelings of hurt, anger, confusion and jealousy, which may become unbearable to deal with and you might find yourself spiralling back into that whirlwind you have just come out of.
Before you either call a friend to fall apart or call him to vent your frustration, take it all in.
Realise that your ex has moved forward and is continuing his life without you.
Don't act: try to allow your thoughts and feelings to pass.
When you first hear news that you are not expecting, it is natural to feel a bundle of mixed emotions, but over a course of time your emotions will change; you will feel differently as the news kicks in.
Yes, it will make you sad to know he has moved on while you are suffering, it is extremely painful to know that he is out there treating another woman better than you and not to mention the obvious: that you are carrying his unborn child.
You are missing out on nothing, a man who is not willing to be a part of his child's life is totally unreliable: he could very easily walk out on anyone, at any time, for any reason.

Abandoned Pregnant

You know what he is really like after all, and any relationship he is in may be built on complete lies.
I mean, honestly: what type of woman would want to be in a relationship with a man who wants nothing to do with his own child? What kind of woman would even want to be with a man who is expecting a baby with someone else?
If she does know about you being pregnant, but simply does not care because she feels it does not involve her then she is just as bad as he is, therefore she is not worth wasting any time on worrying about what she thinks of you based on whatever your ex has told her.

There is a saying: "The only person worse than a dead beat dad is the woman he is with."

Avoid desperate attempts trying to contact her to explain your side of things, even if you find out your ex has told her the baby isn't his.
I would not advise that you go out of your way to inform this woman of anything she doesn't know either: avoid any drama at all costs! Sadly, you will end up looking the fool if you do confront her as your ex has made it clear he does not want to be with you.
There are so many awful things happening in the world, don't put yourself and your unborn child at risk of anyone who could potentially cause you harm.

Abandoned Pregnant

As horrible and disgusting as the subject I am moving on to is, I do want to talk about it because it does happen.

If you discover your ex is having another baby with a woman who happens to be pregnant at the same time as you, then you must not allow her being pregnant to annoy you. I know it is hard.
This is going to sound harsh, but this woman's pregnancy has nothing to do with you.
You can't stop your ex from getting anyone else pregnant just because you are.
You cannot expect him to behave in a certain way because you feel it is the right thing for him to do. Based on his actions, from the way he has treated you, you are clearly setting yourself up for disappointment.
It is an upsetting situation, yet this woman and the baby she is having aren't your responsibility, so you shouldn't worry about her pregnancy or whatever she is doing.
Besides, when you have your baby you will be so wrapped up in him or her that you won't even have time to become annoyed by this woman's situation anymore.
Your ex has caused you enough pain as it is, pregnancy can cause havoc on our bodies - especially in the first few months - so don't take on any more stress from his new interest, who is none of your business.

This happened to me, during my second pregnancy several people informed me that my ex had got

Abandoned Pregnant

someone else pregnant and her due date was not too far behind mine.

Needless to say, the hurt and disgust I felt was immense.

I could not believe it.

I was told that like me, he had left this woman pregnant. During an argument with my ex, I asked him about this other woman; he denied her existence to me, said there was no baby and that if he didn't want to have a baby with me, why would he be having another baby with someone else? I did not believe him though, as I had found out he had also denied my pregnancy to people he didn't want to know.

I did not make any attempts to try to discover the identity of this other woman, nor was I interested in trying to find out anything else. Sure, I was curious about things – such as how long he had been seeing her etc. – but I just knew I had to forget about them both.

I had to let him make his own decisions and then he could live with his choices.

You too, also have to live with your own choices.

You may not like to hear this but it is true, when we are in a relationship with a man, or sexually involved with him, he becomes a 'potential father' to your children.

That is a choice you have made whether you were aware of it or not.

A woman knows deep down if the man she is seeing is wrong for her; but she may still turn a blind eye to all the warning signals that give the biggest signs that it will only end in disaster.

It can feel as if your whole world has come crashing down around you if the father of your baby denies his paternity. It is very frustrating, especially when you 100% know he is the father.

Getting a reluctant man to recognise that he truly is a child's biological father is far from an easy task; a paternity test can easily settle the question, but even so, the biological proof does not make a father.

For your ex to deny his paternity, just to get out of his responsibilities, is a cruel and hurtful thing to do to you at such a vulnerable time in your life.

Sadly, a lot of men do this.

There are lots of other reasons why your ex could be claiming he isn't your baby's father; he may believe that he really isn't the father, he could be trying to buy himself some time as he may not be ready to have a baby, or he could already have a family.

Getting your ex to do a DNA test could be difficult: if you suggest a test, he might refuse, leaving you with no way of proving your baby is his - which is one of the reasons why he may deny your child in the first place.

If the father of your child does this, you could always go through the Child Maintenance Service once you have had your baby: they will seek financial support for your child from him and if he denies his paternity the agency will arrange DNA tests for him, you and the baby.

If he refuses to cooperate, or does not turn up for the DNA test, then the Child Maintenance Service will presume your ex to be the father, he will then be made to make a monthly financial contribution out of his monthly wages, (considering he has a job) towards his child's life.

If your ex is in receipt of benefits, it will be deducted from whatever he receives.

Again, the advice regarding the Child Maintenance Service depends on whether you reside in the UK, but the US has a very similar system.

If you do not want to go down this route then you may find it extremely hard to get any sort of evidence that your ex is indeed the father of your child. If you lived together at the time you conceived and can prove it by providing proofs such as council tax bills with both your names on it; his paternity can also be presumed by the Child Maintenance Service that way.

You could just leave it up to him to establish paternity, meaning he has to put forth the effort to take you to get paternity testing done.

But be prepared for this not to happen!

Unfortunately, there is nothing that you can do to force a man to be a father. If you know for sure that your ex is the father of your child and you have not been with anybody else apart from him around the time you conceived, then it really doesn't matter what he thinks or what he might tell people.

Abandoned Pregnant

You're bound to feel humiliated if other people believe his claims are true and you might even try to defend yourself, but why waste your time?
Karma has a funny way of dealing with these things.
Your child may look just like him (unfortunately for you) to the point that everybody who knows his/her father notices the resemblance.
Both my exes have told me in anger during both my pregnancies that they were not the fathers of my children, it really ate at me inside especially as I knew their claims were ridiculous.
Deep down they knew that they were the fathers to my children but said these things to hurt me.

Chapter 5
Dealing With Rejection

It hurts, I know from first hand experience, having dealt with it twice.
Rejection.
It's horrible, especially when it's not just you being rejected, but also your baby, who is a part of that man who is rejecting you both.
You can't understand why he would do this to you, you think back to all the things you ever did for him or to help him out, and wonder how on earth he manages to sleep at night treating you and his baby the way he does.
The simple explanation why is because the fun has stopped and now you have responsibilities. Parenting is hard work and your ex has chosen to run away.
Feeling rejected is enough to make anyone angry and upset, but being rejected by the father of your child is just awful. It can make you feel like you are nothing, when in fact he is the one who is just that: nothing. He had a choice to be a father to his child but instead has chosen not to do anything.
You, on the other hand, are the strong one who has made the decision and stuck to it to give life to your child under these circumstances; because deep down you know you can do it without your ex, you don't need him.

Abandoned Pregnant

I know what it's like when your mind can't help thinking about other women you know, who were fortunate enough to choose men who have stuck around in theirs child's life, and you feel like an idiot but you mustn't cover yourself under any flaws to justify why your ex has rejected you.

When you first discovered that you were being rejected by the father of your child during your pregnancy, I would not be surprised if you threw up. That feeling is enough to make you physically sick and could even drag you into depression, especially if you didn't speak to anyone and keep in your feelings you could suffer from side effects and symptoms of rejection such as being unable to eat anything, not sleeping at night, staying in bed all day.

Another reason you are feeling so bad right now, as you're rejected by the father of your child, is that you believe your worth or value is solely determined by his opinion of you, which is not true.

Don't allow ex to make you acknowledge false facts about yourself: it can result in you having false beliefs about who you really are.

Don't add to your suffering by being hard on yourself: self-blame only feeds the rejection, as you will basically be rejecting yourself. Kicking yourself when you are already down will only make things much worse.

It is quite common for people who have been rejected to become more critical with themselves.

Abandoned Pregnant

You need to remember that all of the intense negative emotions you are feeling are temporary, and that you might even be thankful for this experience in the future. Rejection happens to everyone at some stage in their life; your age, background, wisdom and skills or how clever you are doesn't matter.

There is only one way to guarantee you will never get rejected and that is by having no sort of interaction with anybody ever again. That is not how you are supposed to live your life.

This probably isn't the first time you've experienced rejection and you will have to accept that it's not going to be the last time either; try to look at it in the right way: you have overcome and defeated this emotion before, so you can and you will defeat it again.

Being rejected by your child's father can make you disconnect from friends and family especially those who are happy in their relationships. That's a part of what rejection does: it can make us feel unsettled in a social or romantic environment.

One way to overcome this is to force yourself to reach out to friends and family to receive emotional support from them, and remind yourself that you are loved, cared for, wanted, and valued.

Connect with all those who you know genuinely care about you and appreciate you.

Self-affirmations are a very good way to restore your confidence. Self-affirmations remind us of our skills, abilities and blessings.

Abandoned Pregnant

Believe that being rejected by your ex has happened for a greater reason. Sometimes when things leave us in distress, it is hard to see why it happened and not acknowledge a higher purpose for what has happened, but that higher purpose always reveals itself in time. In the future, you might even be happy and grateful to your ex that he rejected you as you may find a new and much better partner. We tend to find love when and where we least expect it.

Chapter 6
Stop Trying To Make Your Ex See Sense

Some women do not want to accept and cannot believe or begin to contemplate the fact that the father of their child really is uninterested in being involved in their child's life.

Many women hold onto hope that they will eventually talk their exes round to the idea before the baby is born and are devastated when this doesn't happen.

Some women even go as far as lying about the health of their baby to try to get some sort of attention or reaction from their ex which is just wrong on so many levels; they may even try explaining all the negative effects an absent father has in a child's life and how important it is for a child to know who their father is. They try to convince him to be a father and plea for an explanation as to why he is acting that way, because they really don't understand he is doing it because he wants to!

Your ex is not going to feel sorry for you and you will only end up being a nuisance to him, which could result in him becoming agitated and doing more hurtful things to you in an attempt to get you to leave him alone. At this point you are like an itch he just cannot scratch.

If your ex is capable of rejecting his own child who knows what else he is capable of; he could be bad mouthing you, or even entertaining his friends with your pain if you have sent him continuous texts or voice messages appearing desperate.

It is upsetting to think about, but there is a chance he and other people around him could be laughing at your expense.

He may lead you on only to intentionally let you down, or to get a reaction out of you.

Do not give him the satisfaction of making you out to be some love sick desperate woman who just can't get over him.

Of course, you know that's not true, all you want is a father for your child but unfortunately most of these types of men don't realise that, they are not even thinking that far ahead, a baby isn't really a reality to them until it is born.

It is important that you stay calm and relaxed; trying to force your child's father into the equation is only going to bring more stress into your life.

Do not waste your time trying to convince this irresponsible man to become involved in his child's life.

No woman should have to come close to begging a man to know his own child: he either wants to or he doesn't.

The game has totally changed now, your ex is no longer a priority in your life, and your baby is.

You may have once believed that this guy was the love of your life, but somehow I really don't think he deserves that title as he is so mixed up and unpredictable.

Abandoned Pregnant

I used to try so hard to convince both my exes during my pregnancies to either come back and we could try to work it out, or at least to remain friends for the sake of our baby. I was so desperate for them to care, I didn't realise I was actually becoming repulsive to them, I was showing them I had lost all my self-respect and pride by literally begging them to do something they didn't want to do, it was like I was telling them I couldn't do it on my own, or without them.

After experiencing rejection from my ex during my first pregnancy, continuous failed attempts in trying to talk him around, and even after he changed his number on me, the truth still never really dawned on me that he really did not have any interest in me or the baby if he was prepared to cut all contact by changing his number.

I did the same thing in my second pregnancy with my ex at that time: I tried and pleaded with him, to make him see what he was doing to me and the affects his actions would have on his child in the future; he didn't care either.

It took me a long time to see what they saw at the time: a desperate woman who didn't understand what "not interested" meant.

I had low self-esteem then and was very vulnerable. Don't do things that you will later regret and end up feeling embarrassed or ashamed about. Women in general make things so much harder for themselves at the end of relationships by not wanting to accept that it's really over; instead we try to win our exes back rather than think of ways to help us move on and not end back up in the same situation.

You are fooling yourself by thinking a conversation or a text will make your ex want to suddenly change his mind and want to take on responsibilities he has tried so hard to avoid, the choice has got to be his.

Why would you want somebody who doesn't really want to be around in contact with your child, somebody who is here because of something you said or did? It is not genuine and your ex may end up resenting or taking it out on your child who really, he didn't want. Children pick up on things very quickly, you don't want your child to feel unwanted or unloved. Sometimes, your ex not being around could be the best thing for you and your child. Your ex could have underlying issues from his childhood that you may not aware of, explaining why he is behaving this way; I know that both my exes had issues with their fathers.

You would think that men who have grown up without having a father would not want the same for their children, but it doesn't always go that way. A lot of men who leave women pregnant have unresolved issues with their parents, or have been raised without a father themselves and they think that because they have managed throughout life without having a dad, so will their child.

They don't think about that child growing up and becoming a woman or a man who he will one day have to face to explain why he was absent in their life.

Abandoned Pregnant

As much as you might want to tell your ex all the possible side effects his behaviour will have on not only your child, but on him in the future there is really no need for you to do that. He is well aware of the choice he has made and all the side effects of his actions. You do not need to point anything out to him. He won't thank you for it, and the last thing he will want to do after you tell him about his actions and the consequences of them, is to do as you say.

Whenever I felt the urge to attempt preaching to my ex again, I reminded myself by reading everything I had written that he had said and done. I reminded myself of the date when I last saw him and as the days would go by, I would tell myself that nobody who cared about me could go this long without knowing how I was doing.

I set my mind up to think a certain way - it was hard at first, but it got easier - I told myself things I would tell a friend in my situation; as often, we are better at giving out good advice than at taking our own.

I listened to the advice I gave myself and decided to follow it as I knew it was good for me. I didn't want to live like that anymore, constantly thinking about my ex and trying to persuade him to be a father to our child; it was emotionally draining and I always ended up feeling like a fool. I would tell myself I wouldn't call or text him again and still end up doing it! It had to stop and I had to take control of my emotions. I wanted to show him I wasn't thinking about him anymore and that I was getting on with my life.

Abandoned Pregnant

I was able to do this by recalling, every time I felt like I wanted to call him that he didn't want to speak to me or he would have called me himself. I sometimes used to get this idea in my head that maybe he really did want to call me but he didn't know how to after being so mean to me, but I now know that if somebody really wants to speak to a person, no matter what has happened, they will make the effort and do whatever it takes to sort things out, especially when it's about something as important as a baby. I realised I could not change my ex's behaviour, but what I could change was how I reacted to him, and my feelings about him.

I was the one who was carrying his baby, I had something for him; he didn't have anything for me, so why was I chasing him?

He knew where I lived and how to contact me if he wanted to.

Chapter 7
Revenge

We have all experienced it, that heated feeling of wanting to punish someone who has caused you pain.
There will no doubt be times when you feel like you need to get revenge on your ex; he has taken liberties in so many ways and just got away with it, you want to teach him a lesson and you want him to feel as angry as you are, or cause him an equivalent amount of stress.
Don't do it.
You will definitely be making things a whole lot worse and your ex will believe his actions towards you are justified because of your behaviour.
You are more than likely the number one person in his life right now who would want to cause him grief, making you also the number one suspect. Should any of his belongings, property, vehicles, etc. be damaged, you can be sure your name will blamed.
The consequences of revenge are often unthought-of. What if someone gets hurt, injured or humiliated to the point of no return? What if that person turns out to be you? Revenge can back fire no matter how well you may think you have planned it. You could get yourself in problems with other people, or even the law.

At the time of seeking revenge it may seem to appear harmless, but acts of revenge can cause serious damage in a person's life; you can end up hurting others who are innocent, or who care about the person.

If you have been telling everybody who knows your ex what a dog he is and about how poorly he has treated you STOP!
Nobody really cares, nobody can change your situation, it isn't their problem and you will only be giving them something to talk or even laugh about with someone else. Don't allow your life to be a topic of discussion for others. As much as you might want to damage your ex's reputation it won't change anything apart from damaging your own reputation in the process. People respect a woman who respects herself; have some dignity and pride, don't embarrass yourself. You are better than that.
Seeking revenge is not just payback, it also shows your ability to handle crisis. You are about to become a mother, so it's best to behave maturely as you will face catastrophes in your life as a parent.
Feelings of revenge are negative energy, which is not good for your mind or health; you really don't have time to be holding onto any bitterness or stress, you have wasted enough time over this guy already.
Which leads me onto why they say living well is the best revenge.
A lot of women think that "living well" simply means to ensure that they look good, be happy and pretend everything is going just great the next time that they bump into their ex.

Abandoned Pregnant

The living well part has nothing to do with your ex, that part is for you. It has nothing to do with your ex knowing how well you are doing without him, it's about you knowing it, knowing that you are happy and not feeling that you need him in your life.
When you hold a grudge, you are the one carrying that weight. Getting revenge doesn't dismiss the behaviour of your ex that hurt you, it just makes the cycle of anger and pain continue. Do not lower yourself to his level, as you then become equally as bad as he is.
Instead of seeking revenge it is better to accept what has happened and try to make peace with the issue; not for your ex, but for yourself.
Replace negative feelings with positive thinking, this will help you to move forward. Cut yourself off from anyone who offends you in ways that you feel you need to seek revenge; you don't need to have any more interaction with these people. Take yourself away from those who have wronged you to the point you cannot get past it and don't ever allow them to see you suffer.
I honestly believe that what goes around comes around, karma is real, we all get back what we give out and your ex's karma may come a lot sooner if you have no part in it and leave it to the universe so that you can have a clean conscience.

I tried to get revenge on both my exes during both of my pregnancies. The father of my first child got off lightly - I think it was because I had the support of his mum, so I would only do petty things to him, like get my

Abandoned Pregnant

friends to prank call him which I knew he found annoying, much to my satisfaction. I would get a huge kick out if it, being a silly teen.
During my second pregnancy, oh boy, did I take things a lot further!
In one day I called about 15 cabs to my ex's mums house, where he lived, I ordered about 12 pizzas from different food outlets that delivered as well ordering from around 8 different Chinese restaurants in the area that also delivered. I registered his email address and mobile number to gay porn websites, I put his mobile number on loan applications and stuff like that so he would receive nuisance calls. I sent long broadcasts around, on blackberry messenger, about him and what he had done to me to the people who knew us, which eventually got around to those who didn't. I heard that one night he got into an altercation outside a club, where someone said to him no wonder why some girl was sending all broadcasts around about him.
Needless to say, at the time I learned of that drama I was very happy; people had seen my messages and had read all about what an evil man he was. I never once stopped to think about how my immature behaviour was making me look as I was too wrapped up in my own anger. All I could focus on was ways to bring my ex down. He was very popular in the area we lived in because of his job so I constantly thought up ways I could shame him, and I did them. I once called up my ex's work place pretending to be a nurse from the GUM clinic who was trying to desperately make contact with

him, I told the man on the other end of the line that my ex had left his mobile and work numbers on the forms, but I couldn't get through to his mobile and it is urgent that I speak with him. I stressed the importance of my call being returned and the man I was speaking to seemed to believe every word I said, he assured me they would urge him to return my call, he sounded absolutely embarrassed and at the time I found it very funny, in fact if I am honest... I still do.
I did other petty and silly things too like expose any secrets I knew about him, and tell others what he had told me about them. I couldn't see what I was doing to my own reputation in the midst of it all.
It was only as time passed that I started to feel embarrassed and ashamed for the way I behaved, but I do also know that my hormones during my pregnancy had a huge part to play in my emotions. It was telling everyone about what he had done to me and that, I regret the most. At the time I was really angry, he was ignoring, avoiding and rejecting me, so I made sure that the people I knew he wasn't avoiding would have plenty to tell him about what I was saying about him; he wasn't going to get me out of sight out of mind so easily.
During the time I was sending the broadcasts on Blackberry Messenger about my ex, he did actually send me a text message telling me to stop doing what I was doing, or I would never get what I wanted. That enraged me further, as I then realised that he cared more about what others though about him than caring about our unborn child.

Abandoned Pregnant

I didn't stop because I was still angry; I then discovered he was responding to all the rumours from my broadcasts about him by saying bad things about me, so I then stopped my broadcasts and he stopped responding to them.
Pretty stupid now I'm looking back on it, I will put it down to being young.

Chapter 8
When will I stop feeling like this?!

With each day that goes by, you may become more aware of exactly how long it has been since you last had contact with your ex; you might find yourself crying everyday just wishing that you could turn back time and do or say something differently to make him stay.
You might hide your true feelings from friends and family because you just feel so lost for words and don't know what to tell them about him anymore. Be honest with them: they will be more understanding upon learning of the way you are being treated.

It's understandable that you just cannot believe the person he turned out to be. You miss him, you think you still love him, then half an hour later you hate him. You know deep down that a man who truly loves a woman or at least cares about her, doesn't treat her this way, but you still can't help wishing that he would change.
You try to make sense of everything in your head over and over again, you may even take some of the blame and say to yourself 'well, he did say he didn't want to have the baby, this was my decision' and you are right; but a real man would not care about the fact that he did not want the baby, a real man would eventually respect your wishes to keep his baby although he may not be

Abandoned Pregnant

happy about it, he realises he has no control over your body, and recognises the fact that he is having a child who he will have to accept responsibility for. You would not have to run down a real man to care about his child, you already know this.

It's not nice going to bed and wake up alone when you have been used to sharing a bed with your partner. The bed may now feel empty and cold without that warmth you used to share, but it's not forever! You will soon have your baby to cradle up to you and to keep each other cosy; that feeling is so much better than sharing a bed with any man.

It's really horrible to have your ex disappear out of your life, much more so when you are having a baby for them; you thought he would be around to help you, and watch his child grow but he's gone and no amount of reasoning you do can make him stay, no matter how desperate you are.

If your ex has been ignoring you I am sure you have tried everything to get his attention but to no avail. How long are you going to allow yourself to mourn over him? You are the only person in control of your feelings, only you can change them.

Everything you are going through is not unusual for a single woman during pregnancy.

I remember what I went through like it happened yesterday. The first time I was left pregnant I was crushed, I felt sick to my stomach that the man whom I loved and had lived with for the past three years could just abandon, ignore and reject me.

I could not believe it, the heartbreak it caused me was indescribable. I so desperately wanted to forget about him, but at the same time I could not get the thought out of my head that he didn't want my baby. I remember one day when I was eight months pregnant, I was walking back from the train station and I saw the father of my child drive past with some girl in his car in the passenger seat; needless to say it made me so angry that night I went to bed I imagined myself doing some pretty evil things to him as I drifted off to sleep. It was no wonder why I dreamt of him so much and why my daughter turned out the splitting image of his side of the family. That day I saw him with the girl in his car, I thought he really didn't love me anymore and this was really it, it was over, I was left on my own with our baby. I never thought we would end up getting back together, but we did and a lot of the worrying and stress I caused myself turned out to be pointless in the end anyway.

With my second time being pregnant and alone I took it so much worse. I had known my ex for over 10 years and never expected he could do this do me; especially as he was around when I was bringing up my daughter alone and he knew how I felt about what my ex had done to me because we had spoken about it.

I found out I was pregnant on Valentine's Day, and I gave birth on 10/10/10. My son is truly a lucky charm; he is smart, clever, handsome and so funny! His father is definitely missing out and it's not my problem, it's his.

Abandoned Pregnant

His mother (my son's grandmother) isn't missil don't care about him anymore, what he does, who he sees, where he goes or how many kids he has... It doesn't bother me.
This is coming from a person who never ever thought they could see a way forward, there was a time during both my pregnancies I just wanted to give up on everything and stay in bed; especially when it happened the second time. I thought to myself am I cursed? Do I not deserve to be happy whenever I'm pregnant? I couldn't see it was because of the choices I made that I ended up in those situations.
You cannot let go of your pain and move forward with your life if you are resisting it, in order to move on you must fully embrace your pain. As difficult as it will be, allow yourself to feel your loss sadness and grief, write down what your feeling and come to terms with the emotions you are going through.
You will only stop feeling as you do when you decide to. You cannot force yourself to overcome these feelings before you are ready to do so. Things happen so fast that you will wake up one morning and later in the evening think 'hang on... I haven't thought about my ex all day!' And you will feel so good about it. Eventually a week will pass where you notice that although you may have thought of him, it was only for a few minutes and you changed your thoughts over to something else. That's how it happens. You're probably thinking you don't see it happening to you, but I assure you it will, in your own time.

Abandoned Pregnant

You can't compare your feelings with someone else's; in other words if you have a friend or know of someone who has been in a situation similar to yours there is no point in asking them how long it took them to get over their ex, as everyone is different. That person you know could have felt differently towards their ex than how you feel about yours, their ex could have behaved differently than yours, and treated her differently than how your ex treated you. Everyone has their own individual circumstances and take different ways and time frames to deal with things; it also depends on whether you seek professional help in addressing your issues.

Chapter 9
Accepting Things As They Are

You probably never thought in all of your life you were going to experience the emotions and pain that this situation has brought you. Sometimes, we think that bad things can't happen to us, only to other people, but that's just not true. Life is unpredictable and things change, nothing is permanent. It goes without saying that what has happened to you will no doubt have an impact on your life, but you need to find the ability to truly accept your circumstances and embrace it.

Whether or not your ex has moved on to a new relationship, or if he is having another baby with someone else, if he is denying your baby is his, or if he is just rejecting all responsibilities towards your child, you need to accept what has happened, you have been though a tough time, dealing with what is branded a 'deadbeat dad.'

Ladies, I personally feel your pain in having to deal with these types of men.

Depending on your situation and the way your ex has treated you, I guess you have a choice to make.

Are you going to cut him out of you and your baby's life completely?

Or are you going to get on with your life, without any expectations from this guy - but if at some point he wants to have contact with his child, then that's a plus, right?

Accepting and coming to terms with your new responsibilities as a single mum can be pretty scary, you will be solely responsible for all of your child's needs.

You will most probably also experience extra financial stress.

It is all so easy to feel resentful and overwhelmed with the situation you are in.

But you must try not to worry, because these things can be dealt with and you will deal with them.

Everything will become easier as you adapt.

Being angry about your situation will only make it harder for you in coping with it, and staying angry won't help you in coming to terms with your new life.

It takes great effort to let go of a failed relationship, the fact you are pregnant as well is bound to make it harder, but you have to learn to heal yourself without allowing those complicated feelings to take over.

Everyone has been hurt or betrayed by someone close to them at a time in their lives, either by words or actions.

These open wounds can leave you with negative feelings like hate, bitterness, anger and vengefulness.

You cannot change the past, but you can apologise, let go, and forgive. Take responsibility for yourself, learn, and change the present and the future by moving forward.

I personally have learned from experience, that if you don't practice forgiveness, you might be the one to end up needing forgiveness the most. Don't act on those lingering negative feelings that you haven't dealt with.

That is why I highly recommend going to see a counsellor for what you have been through.

What has happened will always remain a part of your life, and you need to learn how to move away from your role as victim and release the control and power that your ex and the situation had in your life.

Whether you choose to grow or to remain a victim is up to you.

Writing down what you have been through gives you a good sense of relief; it helps to unleash your thoughts and feelings.

It's also how this book came together.

Whether it's in the notes section of your phone, handwritten on a notepad, or on your laptop, the act of writing can help you to let off steam.

Also, if your ex is still on any of your social media accounts like Facebook, then remove him.

Something as simple as seeing a picture of him being happy with a status like 'Life is good' has the ability to change your mood completely, or if you see a new woman who likes all his pictures you could easily become obsessed with trying to find out who she is, which is all pointless because it's not going to change anything apart from your feelings going back into whirl wind mode.

If you find that the situation is still really bothering you then speak to a counsellor, or a friend that you can trust, if you want someone to help you make sense of things and give you a clearer view.

You should probably think yourself lucky your ex has gone; one of the benefits to come out of your situation is that you won't get caught up in ex-sex.

So many women find it hard to stop being intimate with the fathers of their children when they are no longer in a relationship allowing themselves to be used and their feelings totally disregarded, resulting in their self-esteem hitting rock bottom.

There are positives to being single, you become more independent and learn more about yourself, you can also develop coping skills, have more time to spend with family and friends and to do the things that you enjoy.

There are also positive sides to being a single mum, like not having anyone to undermine your authority, not having to consider the fathers opinion in anything to do with your child, and not having to share your child during the weekends and holidays.

It took me some time to accept things as the way they were in both of my pregnancies, especially my first. I really struggled and I found it upsetting when I had to build my baby's cot by myself at eight months pregnant; all I could think of was how my ex could be so horrible to leave me to do these things alone. I imagined how that moment should have been, I pictured the father of my child putting up our baby's cot while I waited excitedly for it to be built, but what I should have done instead was pat myself on the back and been proud that

Abandoned Pregnant

I was able to put my baby's cot up by myself. I should have celebrated the fact that I did not need my ex, but I was too angry at the time to see any positive sides to my situation.

It was hard to see myself as a single mum because I never saw it coming - but who does!
What was even harder to accept was the rejection from my ex. I kept feeling like it was something I had done wrong and thought I could fix it, but in the end I realised that they were his issues not mine.
I was a lot happier, more calm and peaceful when I accepted everything instead of constantly battling, trying to change things.
Why waste time attempting to change things you cannot when there are so many things that you can change? You can change your appearance, your hair, the way you dress, your behaviour, how you respond to the behaviour of others, the friends you keep, the choices you make, the responsibility you take for yourself and who you choose to blame, the way you communicate with others, the place you live, work... I could go on.

Acceptance is a choice, a hard one definitely, but in the end it's a choice that only you can make for yourself at any given situation in your life.
Accepting things does not mean you are weak or that you are allowing yourself to be walked over, it just

Abandoned Pregnant

means that you are moving on from whatever happened.

Chapter 10
Learning From This Experience

With everything you have been through, it is probably right for me to assume that you have gotten some sort of wakeup call from this experience, and learned a lesson in what you should do and don't do in relationships, and out of them.

A wake up call is a message that things are not ok and that change is necessary, usually by the time you are aware of your calling, things have already turned into a full blown crisis.

When you run into a crisis it can be a turning point where you make a change, either for the better or for the worse in your life.

A wake up call can also be an opportunity to try to fix that crisis and make things right – if it isn't too late to do so.

You may have arrived at a point of truth in your life, where you finally come to grasps with your situation and realise that you and your little one deserve better.

Maybe you have decided to never ever put yourself in these chaotic circumstances again.

Some wake up calls don't always come to us as a shock; usually there have been blatant hints along the way which have been ignored.

Abandoned Pregnant

Being away from your ex for a while can suddenly give you an outside look into the relationship and finally you get to see what other people saw in him and realise why none of your friends or family members may not have liked him.

Maybe during your relationship, you neglected friends and put your ex before existing friendships, so now you don't have the same number of friends that you started out with at the beginning of your relationship with this guy; these things do happen.

You might have put your ex before family members and not have been there for someone special in your life, who really needed you because you were too busy being wrapped up in him.

Now you have discovered what he is really like you may start to remember these things and feel angry with yourself or even regret your choices.

The damage has already been done, but it does not mean that you can't or shouldn't apologise to the people whose feelings you may have hurt.

You are bound to feel embarrassed, but if these people really do care about you then they will sympathise with your situation and accept your apology.

Women can do really stupid things when they believe that they are in love, and other women should be able to relate to that feeling and be there for each other when we need a friend to lean on and to talk to.

You may think over how desperately you behaved to try to get your ex's attention during your pregnancy while he was ignoring you and feel ashamed, but what

matters now is that you recognise this behaviour was inappropriate and you moved on.
Part of your wakeup call will include acknowledging all those signs you ignored in your relationship with your ex, think back to a time where he made that insulting comment you didn't like or when his actions appeared to come across as dodgy.
Revisit those moments and be honest with yourself.

It's time to take action, you can dramatically change the negative energy in your life, and it doesn't take that long for you to be able to see the results. Positive energy attracts more positive energy and the same goes for the opposite terms. Evaluate your life, write down your new intentions, list everything and everyone that is bringing you down and your priority is to then clear the clutter, physically and mentally. This includes any house work, errands, bills to sort out, appointments or conversations that you are avoiding.
Decide on how many of these things you can complete and set yourself a deadline.
Challenge yourself, but also be realistic about the things that you can complete, prioritise your list in terms of how much positive energy you will lose when you think about them, you will be amazed at how many you will be able to cross off. You can decide on whether you want to make new lists that are manageable, but if we think that we have to change our lives forever, that can become overwhelming.

Abandoned Pregnant

Make a commitment to yourself and take action, it is important to build up your positive energy day by day.
Do something that makes you happy and reward yourself for a job well done.
Only you know what will make you feel fulfilled and satisfied, when you want to achieve a goal I seriously stress and recommend that you always write it down, and check to see how much work you have achieved towards it every day.
Visualise the best possible outcome you would like to happen in your life, hold on to that image, and that feeling, work towards having that future and don't hold yourself back. Consistency is the key, start early and give each milestone the time it needs. Try to stay motivated, read up quotes by people you are inspired by, or listen to music that gives you that boost you need. Create an environment where you can thrive.
Recreate your life story, only you can change the script. One of the hardest things to do is look our demons straight in the face and admit their existence to ourselves. Stand in front of your mirror on your own and honestly tell yourself what you are afraid of, what you regret, and what you are ashamed of.
It might be unpleasant and scary because when we say things out loud, they become real. But this is a good thing because once you've identified your inner clutter, you can begin to alleviate it. We cannot fight off phantom demons, make them real and then kick them where the sun doesn't shine.
Believe in yourself.

Abandoned Pregnant

Chapter 11
Letting Go

It can be so tempting to try just one more time at attempts in making the father of your child become interested in the baby he does not want.
Don't do it. You will only be setting yourself up for more upset and heartbreak which you really don't need now while you have a new-born to look after.
This is the time you should be bonding with your child, don't let your ex distract you from it.
Your baby will sense something is not right with you if you are angry or irritated and it could interfere in your bonding, resulting in a crying baby.
You have tried to get your ex involved in his child's life; the more you push him to be a father, the more you are in fact pushing him away. He is probably annoyed that you haven't got the message and is wondering when you will forget about him and move on.
Assuming he knows how to contact you, it is now up to you to leave it to your ex to show you that he wants to be in his child's life.
It is time to let go and move on with your life.
If you have brothers, uncles or close male friends they can be father figures for your child.
My uncle has been a father figure to me all my life, he has been there for me all the times - a real man would

be there for his child - and the love I have for him is not as a niece should love her uncle, but as a daughter should love her father.

He has bailed me out of every major crisis in my life, including financial ones and most importantly, he is a positive role model who has set a great example of what a real man is and I am so lucky to have had his support growing up.

If you should have a son but you lack male influence in your life, as he gets older you could enrol him into activities where there are male instructors who will give him a positive male role model.

When you first hold your baby, you will become overwhelmed by such a love you never thought could exist.

You may feel the urge to send you're ex a picture of your new-born, especially if you see any resemblance in your baby that reminds you of his or her father; it may get you thinking about him again.

You might even go through times where you stare at your baby asleep (every mother does it!) and feel sad that this innocent, sweet baby may never know his or her father.

You might think that by sending you're ex a picture of your new-born, he will think to himself 'aww how cute, he or she looks like me, I want to be his or her daddy now.'

I'm sorry but he won't.

Abandoned Pregnant

You sending him a picture of your baby is making him face a reality he really doesn't want to; his worst nightmare in fact, what he has been running from for the past nine months, and as bad as it sounds you would get a better relation out of him with curiosity.
Not knowing what his baby looks like, or not knowing anything about him or her, will be on your ex's mind.
Even though he makes out he doesn't care he will most certainly be curious.
If you do send him a picture of your baby, you will be easing a part of his curiosity, and he doesn't deserve it.
One of the reasons single mums fail to understand why the father of their child does not feel anything towards their cute, sweet, innocent little baby, is because these men have not bonded with the child as you have.
He doesn't know what he is missing out on.
If your ex does try to make contact after hearing you have had the baby, then it is down to you whether you would like to speak to him or not;
But I would like you to bear in mind that he has put you through a lot and you will have come a long way.
After having a baby, a lot of women suffer with post-natal depression, try to stay away from anything stressful and give yourself time to adjust to your new routine in your life as a parent before taking on any issues with your ex.
If he would like to see the baby and you allow him to, then make sure he understands he has one chance and he is either in all the way or out, don't accept any mixed signals; try to have someone there with you and avoid

Abandoned Pregnant

getting into a discussion with him unless it concerns your child.

My ex met my first child when she was six months old, and we eventually got back together when she turned one.
At first it was great, but we had too many unresolved issues from the past and our relationship broke down. Things moved too quickly - I simply accepted his apology, took him back and forgot about everything he had put me through.
At that time I had no respect for myself, no self-love. I now understand why people say never to reconcile with an ex for the sake of your children, because you could end up making them unhappy.
Our relationship lasted for two years.
He is still in our daughter's life.

After my relationship with my daughter's father broke down, about a year later - when I realised we weren't going to get back together - I got back with the very same ex I had left when I decided to reconcile with my daughter's dad.
He completely changed.
He wanted to continue to be with me but dismiss any talk about our baby, it angered me so much that he could actually behave like that.
I could not believe this was the same man who used to say we were like Bonnie & Clyde; we had got up to so

Abandoned Pregnant

much mischief together in our teenage years and shared so many memories together. I thought I would go out of my mind when he started to ignore me during the middle of my pregnancy, I couldn't understand how he cut me off for so long without missing me.

We were so accustomed to speaking to each other for hours every day and I couldn't believe he wasn't missing all the stuff we used to do together.

Chapter 12
Love Yourself

Whether or not you believe it, unless you love yourself, nobody is going to love you and the same thing goes for if you don't respect yourself.
I know this from experience.
Obviously, we would all like to love ourselves but sometimes it's just not that easy; we have to learn how to.
In learning to love ourselves, we then become capable of being loved, and then we are capable of loving others.
Celebrate your past, be proud of yourself that you have got through it all - everything that happened in the past has made you who you are today so embrace it; without it, you wouldn't be you.
We all make mistakes in life, all of us, it doesn't matter who you are, and nobody is perfect.
Let go of any mistakes you have made, learn what you can from them and move on.
Change your outlook on things, your mind-set could have gotten used to thinking one way, you have to transform it and believe that you are worthy of being loved and respected.
You have to seek out the positive things in your life and lift yourself up.

If you don't do it for yourself, nobody else will do it for you.

When you really start to love yourself deeply, you start to feel alive and the people you meet treat you differently.

By loving yourself, the people you come into contact with will respect you more.

Stop all the self-criticism, your imperfect body, your character flaws, your failures and mistakes.

STOP IT!

We don't realise that we have everything we need to be happy with ourselves; quite often we're so scared of being happy that we keep on just waiting for things to change instead of recognising only we can make those changes.

When you do love yourself enough to make those necessary changes, your life will transform almost instantly.

You need to be brutally honest with yourself as you cannot begin to love yourself remaining in the same cycle of denial that we tend to live in when it comes to facing difficult stuff in life that we just don't want to deal with.

Staying in a bad relationship or wanting to reconcile with someone who treats you badly over and over again, is about a lack of self-love and self-respect. Love yourself enough to not try to put things back together.

Forgive yourself for any bad choices you made in the past; you are now growing and changing.

Abandoned Pregnant

Be kind to your mind, if negative thoughts run through your head, gently change those thoughts and don't get angry with yourself for having the thoughts in the first place. Listen to your ideas, do you ever find yourself ignoring your instincts or avoiding your gut feeling? Don't do that anymore, if you want to love yourself, you have to believe in yourself, you have to trust yourself.
Recognise that your thoughts and ideas are valid and you don't always have to act on your ideas, but you should listen to them.
Be patient and kind to yourself, take care of your body.
Enjoy yourself, think back to the things you enjoyed doing or watching as a child and reintroduce them into your life. I know some people don't like to boast about themselves, but you know what? I think it's ok to say how great you are every once in a while. It is ok to admit that you did an amazing job at accomplishing something you never thought you could.
Celebrate yourself, love yourself, do it now.
It is so important that you do this, as some of the things you do will also rub off onto your children as they grow older and I am sure you want them to be happy in their lives. Children's first teachers are their parents, the level of self-respect you model will be the pattern and example that your child is taught. When you show and feel respect for yourself, your child is being taught how to feel about themselves. The more children are around people who have high self-respect or people who feel good about themselves, the more those children will learn to love themselves; happiness comes from within.

Abandoned Pregnant

We teach our children how to be treated by others, and we teach other people how to treat us, getting people to like you is not important, what is important is that you like yourself.

Respect is earned, not given.
Having respect is to have pride and knowledge of your own worth and to value yourself. Self-respect reflects the level of love that we have for ourselves.
It is very easy to confuse self-respect with ego, these two words are not very different in their meanings either. Self-respect is the respect that you have for yourself, while ego is your understanding of your own importance. Self-respect comes first, when you respect yourself and believe in yourself. Then comes your ego, which helps you to realise just how important and special you are. If you have no self-respect for yourself in front of someone, then you cannot have an ego around them.
Even people with high self-respect can start to lose it without realising it. It usually starts with small things, like when you feel put down by a partner or a friend - especially in front of someone else.
If your ex made you feel stupid or dumb, that's a subtle sign that he was subconsciously trying to undermine you and take control, even if he wasn't intentionally trying to. When you start to feel like your partner or a friend is better than you, that's when your self-respect starts to drop around them. You feel a constant need to

please them, just to feel deserving of their attention and affection.

Having love and respect for yourself gives you a better life. You may not realise this, but self-respect will make everyone take you more seriously. Partners and friends will respect you more and love you better.

You will feel more important and mentally stronger which will eventually bring the admiration and respect of others. People who were taking you for granted will subconsciously take you more seriously and treat you like a superior or an equal instead of treating you like a pushover because they will be intimidated by how much self-respect you have for yourself.

It's not easy to gain self-respect and it will not happen overnight.

But if building your self-respect could give you a better life isn't it worth a try?

Chapter 13
Moving On

Many women get themselves into relationships before they are emotionally and mentally ready.
Some women do it out of fear of being alone, some don't like their single status, etc.
Taking time out at the end of a relationship to get to know yourself again can help you in finding the right partner.
Before you are ready to move on to a new relationship, you need to be able to be happy in your own company to avoid entering and accepting a relationship with just anyone.
You also need to be able to look back on your relationship with your ex honestly in order to prevent the same mistakes from happening again, admit responsibility in whatever parts you played as when couples have problems the cause is usually not one sided, you both had a role to play in creating the problem whether it be lack of communication, distance, etc.
You should also be able to really see your ex for who he was in your relationship; love is blind, especially in the beginning, when everything is great.
All of us carry our own baggage from our pasts, none of us want to carry that baggage into a new relationship, nor would we like to get into a relationship with

someone who is carrying baggage. The past isn't the past if it's in your mind, messing up your future.

When you start dating, it should always be because you are ready to and want to, not because of social pressure around you.

Even though you may feel ready to start a new relationship, the thought of actually getting yourself out there may be a bit daunting and off putting, especially when you have become used to being on your own, or if it has been a while since you last went out on a date. You probably won't know where to begin, if you are not one for internet dating or organised events such as speed-dating, then try to start building up your social life. Join a course or gym etc. Most single mums are pushed for time and child care, but it is crucial that you take time to yourself once in a while, to reconnect with the outside world and to enjoy uninterrupted adult conversations.

Moving forward with your life is not just about entering new relationships, it's also about getting to know you, and choosing the things that really matter. Don't let your old problems punish your dreams. Teach yourself how to start choosing the right perspective in your life - for example when you are faced with either being stuck in traffic or standing in a long line at the bank, you have two choices: you can get frustrated and angry, or you can view it differently in a more positive way as life giving you some time off from rushing. The first choice will not be good for you.

Abandoned Pregnant

Moving on is also about breaking away from old habits, activities, and places that you were familiar with when you were with your ex. Change your lifestyle.
If you both used to live together before he left, redecorating can be a great first step towards change; your ex may have also taken a load of stuff with him, so you may have had to make some improvements anyway.
The thought of making such a big change, finalising you are in fact moving on, can be a scary one, but there are good points to redecorating after a break up.
You get to make what used to be 'our' bedroom 'your' bedroom.
You can make it cosy and create a new atmosphere and a different scent.
Getting rid of old bedding you once shared is also a must. Replace everything, pillows, your duvet, all the bed sheets and pillow cases.
Try to choose different patterns and designs that you wouldn't normally when purchasing your new bedding.
Think of it as getting rid of the evidence he was once there.

I lived with the father of my first child when I was pregnant; we had rented a place together and when our relationship ended, he was so angry and mean to me because I had chosen to keep our baby I could no longer live with him while trying to find somewhere else to live. I ended up having to move in with my mum for three months when I was a month into my pregnancy; when I was four months gone, I stayed in a hostel for two months, after that I was then housed by the council.

During the time I was living at my mum's, it was really rough for me. Not only did I have to leave my new job, but I also suffered from severe morning sickness, and missed the place I had called home with my ex; and of course I missed seeing my ex everyday too. I missed our jokes, our talks, waking up to him, everything. There were days I didn't even want to get out of bed. I couldn't sleep at nights and I would often end up falling asleep on the train, on the lengthy journey down from my mum's house to the council in the borough of where my ex and I had resided together.

I was so stressed out and I recall thinking to myself often "when would this nightmare end."

Time really is a great healer. And the mind is a very powerful thing. I had no choice but to motivate myself to carry on doing all the things I needed to do in order to get to that place where I would be ok; and the nightmare ended eventually. My motivation paid off in the end, when I got accepted onto the council's housing list and knew I would soon have somewhere for my baby and I to call home.

Once I was settled into an apartment, I made it mine slowly. I was very lonely at first but then I spent time with myself, something I hadn't gotten around to do in years.

Abandoned Pregnant

I remember feeling so miserable sitting in my kitchen one day; I was close to my due date at that time, my brother and I were speaking about my situation and he told me how sad it mad him to see me like that, that I didn't deserve it, that one day my ex would regret it and that there was nothing worse than living with regrets.

It made me sad to see my younger brother emotional and it made me angry that my ex had hurt my brother by hurting me. That day I realised that what my ex had done to me affected others who cared about me, so I put in tremendous effort into moving on.

I spent hours reading books, educating myself, watching things on the internet, talking to friends on the phone uninterrupted. I was starting to get used to living in my own; I realised that I also enjoyed my space and privacy, something I had not experienced. I had never lived on my own before and I beginning to get comfortable with it. There were times I wished he was there with me but whenever those thoughts entered my mind I would make the decision to think of something else, and I did. I would get so caught up in thinking of that something else my mind would actually wonder onto another subject and I would forget all about him.

Chapter 14
What Do You Tell Your Son Or Daughter About Daddy?

When a very young child asks about their absent father, it is best to keep it simple and general.
You could say something along the lines of, 'sometimes when mummies and daddies don't get along, they decide that everybody will be happier if they stay apart,' or something like 'some children live with just their mums.' Then you can ask your child if they have any questions about what you have just explained, try to be honest with your answers and keep it age appropriate. You could also write a story for your child and again, ask if they have any questions afterwards. Your child's age and maturity will depend on what you say about the situation.
As your child grows, so will your discussions.
A small child's worries are so simple that the last thing we want to do is project our own not-so-simple worries onto them.
It is important to provide some kind of explanation as to why the child's father is absent, so that your child knows it wasn't because of he or she, or something he or she did.
If you can, try to share positive memories of happy times with your ex, as these will become the pieces that your child uses to build up an impression of who he is; something that your child will most likely consider as he

or she grows older and wants to find out more about who they are as a person. Don't talk negatively about your child's father in front of him or her as tempting as it may be: if they hear you talk about how worthless their father is, they might conclude that part of them is worthless too.

Remind your child that you love them unconditionally and that you will always be there for them, do not tell a lie to protect your child's feelings, tell the truth. Give your child reassurances that they are going to be ok without their dad.

Please don't tell your child their dad is dead if he is in fact alive, as children resent their mum when they grow older and they find out the truth, which they will.

Children will start to become very curious about their fathers as they get older; you may need to remain patient as the questions will probably never entirely stop.

If the child asks where their father is, it's ok to tell them that you don't know, don't discourage or be offended by your child's loyalty to their father, as they will use it against you and throw it in your face when they grow up.

Don't try to overcompensate for the absent father, as you will end up with a spoilt child who cannot handle disappointment.

The horrible undeniable truth is that disappointment is a part of life and it makes us stronger, teaches us lessons and adds to our knowledge.

Abandoned Pregnant

If you move on to another relationship and your partner has cared for your child since they were very young, it is not uncommon for him to be seen as the child's birth parent by the child and by others.
Before deciding if you will explain to your child that your partner is not their biological father, you will need to consider a number of things – such as the needs and rights of the child, what your partner thinks, any legal, medical issues, the effect of not telling your child and somebody else doing so at some time instead, and your own thoughts.
If you do decide to tell your child the truth, it is best to tell them when they are young so that they grow up knowing. This helps the knowledge to be less drastic. Try to avoid asking your child to keep the information private as it could cause him or her to feel ashamed or guilty.
You could also put together a scrap book explaining the story of how you got to where you are, your family, your life, your children, your work and your currently partner.
Ideally you and your partner should tell your child together.
You can refer to your ex by their name, or as your child's birth father or biological father. Try to time it sensitively. There are bound to be string reactions, you will need to listen to your child and take notice.
There may be a withdrawal or a lack of reaction, good or bad behaviour; both, could be ways of them coping with the news.

Abandoned Pregnant

Give your child lots of opportunities to express their feelings, your child's life will have permanently changed by the information. Remember, the consequences of keeping a secret are worse than revealing the information.

My son asks me about his father and why he doesn't have one, when his sister does. I can't express how that makes me feel but I have explained to him that mummy and daddy are much happier when they don't speak, that it doesn't mean daddy doesn't love him or care about him, but mummy loves him and will always be there for him, no matter what.

It's so heart-breaking to have to say these things to little innocent children who have done nothing to deserve to be treated this way by their fathers.

I remember as a teenager finding out my biological father did not want me; the feeling was absolutely gut wrenching and I couldn't help thinking about what I had done wrong for him to not care about me.

I was about fourteen years old then and it affected me massively, I would have hated to find that out at a younger age. We need to protect our children from this type of pain, it will cause them to have issues in their adult lives if the situation is not handled properly.

Chapter 15
New Relationships

When you meet a new potential partner - which at some point, you will - you should experience a completely different relationship to any others you have had in the past, as you now have a child.
Please do not become involved with a married man or one who already has a girlfriend; not only is it wrong, but you will be putting yourself at risk to gradually lead right back to where you just came from, having a baby alone.
Don't mess with anyone who is in a relationship, as it never ends well, someone always ends up hurt and that person is more than likely to be you. Even if he promised to leave his girlfriend for you, he probably won't do it; and if he does, then just remember that the way he left her to be with you could be the way he would leave you to be with someone else.

When you do meet someone you feel you enjoy being around, before rushing into a relationship with him, ask yourself, how well do I really know this man?
 It doesn't matter if you have a mutual friend, anyone can put on a mask. A good way to get to know someone is to try to spend time with them when they are around their family; people change in the comfort of their families. Your partner should treat you like the people they already love. Try to avoid speaking in great detail

about the whole situation with your ex. This is something that you do not want being thrown in your face, should things ever turn sour between the two of you.

You must be able to really know that you can truly trust someone over a period of time before you start to share your private business with them. Don't trust someone until you know them.

Your child must come first in any relationship and this is something you should have made your partner understand and be aware of before anything between you even start, although this goes without saying.

It is even more important your child knows that he or she will always come first too; they should not feel threatened in any way by the presence of a new man your life.

Some women are so happy to be in love again - or what they at least think is love - that they neglect their child, putting their new boyfriend's needs first instead.

If you don't want your kids to resent you or have feelings of hatred towards you and have emotional problems now and later on in life because of a lack of love received from you, then don't ever put a man before your child.

Believe me, you will be making the biggest mistake of your life: your child will never be able to love you as they once did, even if they end up forgiving you, and you can bet your life on it: by then that man will be long gone.

Abandoned Pregnant

Don't let your child see you with different men as they grow up either as they will never respect you.
It's not worth it.
If a man sees you are putting him before your own child, you'd better believe he will be calling all the shots in your home in no time – if he isn't doing so already.
You have given him permission to do so without even realising it.
It may have been a while you had some romance in your life, but don't forget where it got you last time; don't let your child see you go through anything like that. Take the time to get to know someone properly before rushing into anything, being friends first is the best way to tell if the friendship can progress.
You can't afford to repeat the same mistakes anymore, you have an example to set now.
You might crave intimacy but respect yourself enough to wait for the right person to come into your life; in the meantime remain focused on raising your child and bettering yourself.
Remember, don't be the woman who needs a man, be the woman a man needs!
When you feel you have found the right partner for you, if he has good intentions he will first and foremost accept that your child will always be your number one priority. He will never complain about it; in fact, he should do the exact opposite and admire and respect you for it.

Abandoned Pregnant

Your new partner should also show an interest in your child's life; after all, he or she is part of you and he is entering their life too.

Any man who does not interact with your child and only shows an interest in you has no intention of sticking around long term and is obviously only after whatever he can get from you.

Becoming involved with men like that, who set out to use you, will only bring out and potentially worsen the abandonment issues you previously suffered from, caused by your ex.

The signs of an insincere man are generally easy to tell, all it takes is common sense and not being in denial to see some of their actions for what they really are.

The first sign you see indicating that things are not going to be ok in your new relationship? Leave.

Don't wait around thinking things will get better and put up with any nonsense because you believe you won't meet anybody else, or that nobody will want to enter a serious relationship with a single mum, because it's just not true and I am sure you know – or have heard of – single mums who have managed to move on and settle down, even going on to get married and having more children.

You can have that too, don't forget that everyone you date becomes a potential husband.

When you first enter a relationship don't have your partner around all the time: you should gradually introduce him into your child's life.

Abandoned Pregnant

Your new relationship will be a big change in your child's life and they will need time to adjust, not to give them that time is unfair.
Your new partner should allow your child to get to know him through events such as a day out at the fun fair, or catching a movie at the cinema etc.
It is a good idea to keep the meeting place neutral and not at each other's houses at first.
Your partner should gradually increase the amount of time he spends with your child.

One evening when my first born was eight months old I was at home with one of my best friends, listening to a funny talk show on the radio. It so happened that her cousin was one of the hosts, and so was my ex.
My friend called the radio station and began to speak to her cousin and informed him that she was with me, her cousin passed this information onto my ex who then asked him to get my number. He called me every day and because he was my ex, who I had shared previous memories with, our conversation flowed as we had nearly three years' worth of catching up to do.
Neither of us had changed much. It didn't take any effort for us to click, we just did.
I felt relaxed speaking with him and being around him, I wasn't as shy as I would have been if I had been dating someone new. We were back together within three months.
He made me laugh and I forgot all about the father of my child, at the time I felt that if he didn't want me

anymore, that was fine because someone else did; my ex. A man's junk was another man's treasure.

Because my daughter was so young at the time, she believed my partner was her father but that changed when her father entered her life.

My ex was very good with my daughter, he treated her as if she was his own, even when he was at work on a break, he would tell me to put her on the phone although she wasn't saying much at that time but he still spoke to her asking her if she was ok and telling her he would see her later. He took an interest in her development and asked questions about her progress in her communication.

There were nights when I would be cleaning up the house and once I was finished I would return to my bedroom to find them both fast asleep on my bed, next to each other. We would go out together, do everything together and whenever we were apart, we would be on the phone to each other; so many people would complain about my phone always being engaged.

We were like a family. I hadn't given the father of my child a second thought, I began to be glad he made his decision and now I was the one who was happy, in a new relationship.

I have recently found out that while I was in my new relationship, the father of my child was hurt that another man was in his daughter's life. He worried my partner could replace him and I believe it was then that he started to have an active role in her life, via his mother.

Abandoned Pregnant

I made a mistake in moving on so quickly, I wasn't really ready for it. The fact that I got back with an ex didn't help things, but I didn't realise it at the time, and because I thought I knew my partner, as he was my ex, from before I got with the father of my first child. I assumed that I didn't need to get to really know him again, but I didn't- really know him; I saw what he wanted me to see.
Of course there were signs that he wasn't the right man for me, but I ignored them anyway because at the time, I felt it was better to overlook them than going back to being alone and feeling like I was going to be single for the rest of my days.
I didn't notice that ignoring these signs was what lead me right back to where I'd started - pregnant and alone again.
I wasn't taking my life seriously yet, and I had no idea of what I wanted; I was just taking whatever came my way day by day and accepted that it was good enough for me. I had no motivation to change my life back then.

Chapter 16
Contact with your ex's family

It is good if you receive any support from your child's paternal side of the family, even if the father himself does not want to be involved, that may just be for the time being; the fact his family has contact with his child will surely at some point create a breakthrough in forming a bond and a relationship in the future.
It can be extremely tough on mothers who have to suddenly form some sort of relationship with members of their ex's family if they haven't known very well – or at all – before their pregnancy.
You don't know what your ex has told them about you, and with them being his family, they are likely to believe him. Do not get into any discussions about your relationship or your break-up with your ex with his family; you could end up getting angry and upset, or even have an argument and making things worse. Whatever you say to his family about him, they are likely to go back and tell him- maybe also adding on things that weren't said or done, especially if they don't like you, so be careful of what – and how much – you say.
Even if his family fill you in on what your ex has said about you and he only told his side of the story, do not feel the need to defend yourself against them, because at the end of the day, like it or not, they will always have

his back – even if he is in the wrong. That's what family is for.

Do not get comfortable and lose focus on what is happening: your ex's family are not your friends, they are your baby's family, and you are responsible for handling the contact with them until your child becomes of age and can manage the relationship himself.
Also, keep your private life exactly that: private.
Whatever you do and whatever is happening in your life is none of your ex's families business, even if they tell you what your ex is up to; it doesn't mean you have to give them any insight into certain areas of your life. You will be so surprised, if things ever turn nasty, how fast things that they shouldn't have known anything about in the first place can be thrown back in your face. Unless it concerns your child, don't tell them your business.
You are going to be in contact with this family for years to come, probably as long as you both live, so you need to start as you mean to continue: how you behave will make all the difference as to how you are treated and respected.
Try not to speak badly about your ex in front of his family, no matter how much you might want to let them know how much of a loser their relative or son is; these people truly love him and you are only going to end up making them not like you, therefore limiting the amount

of support you receive and they will think that you are not over your ex.

If he is bad mouthing you to his family and you are also bad mouthing him to them, they will more than likely not view you both as bad as each other: they'll understand your ex's dislike for you, especially if you are disrespectful to them too. Keep the relationships separate, don't take out any emotions you have stored up for your ex out on his family; just don't mention his name full stop and if they bring him up in conversation, simply say you would rather not speak about him. Stick to the matter at hand, their involvement with your baby. Show your ex's family that your child is your priority.

The most likely person as a source of support is the father of your child's mother; she is after all your son's or daughter's grandmother. If she supports and stands by you during the times you needed her son the most, whether she likes you or not, then she deserves to have an active role in your child's life as their grandmother.

There are some single mothers who get along fine and without any problems with their child's paternal grandmother, but there are others who say that having to deal with their ex's mum is worse than having to deal with their ex!

Paternal Grandmothers can behave very harshly when they want to or when something is happening in their grand child's life that they don't like, that they have no control over; for example if their grandchild's mother got a new boyfriend they don't like. That's why it is important to set the standard as to how you are treated and respected from the very beginning. Your ex's mother should not be able to feel comfortable enough to comment on your private life; you are the person who needs to ensure that there is that line that is not to be crossed, firmly but politely.

Letting off some steam directed at your ex in front of his mother is the number one mistake you can make, as she is the first person who will feel hurt and insulted by any negative comments you make about her son, and while she may allow one or two insults you make to slide, you can be sure she will not forgive anymore and slowly but surely, she will start to dislike you. Your ex's mum already knows her son has let you down, she knows you must be hurt and angry, but you need to behave maturely or I can guarantee you she will soon share similar thoughts as her son, as to why he is no longer around.

If you play your cards right having your child's paternal grandparents in their life can not only be a blessing to your child, but a blessing to you too, as you'll receive extra support. Yes, there will be times when grandma will over advise your ears off or preach about the best way to raise a child, but those are also blessings, as these are the times you when really learn something passed down from an older generation. Pay attention to what is being said now more than ever, as it concerns the upbringing of your child.

Abandoned Pregnant

If you have tried to get your ex partners family to become involved and take an interest in your child but they are not interested, that can really, really hurt. But you have to ask yourself: if they want nothing to do with an innocent baby who is their flesh and blood, what type of people are they toward those who they care about?

Believe it or not there are some mothers out there who do not care about their grandchildren and they go by whatever their son tells them about that child; for example claiming it's not his.

If the mother has never met the woman of her son's child, it can be even harder for her to accept.

I'm

Chapter 17
Contact With Your Ex

If at any time the father of your child should come to his senses and want to become involved in your son's or daughter's life, it is up to you whether or not you allow him to be.
I guess that depends on just how badly he treated you during your pregnancy. It may take some time before you are able to speak to him again, after everything that has happened. I know that if the father of my son contacted me, I would certainly not be able to speak to him right now, as I would be angry. It took him so long to care, although others might look at it as "well, at least he's made contact now and not never," but it's really not just as simple as that. You start to wonder: "is this man going to set a good example in my child's life? If he can treat me so badly during my pregnancy with his baby what's to say he won't do it again? Is he committed to being a father now or will he be in and out of my child's life?"
It's scary. Especially when you have come so far without him, the last thing you need is to have him back in your life, causing you grief and drama.
At the same time you want what's best for your child, you want he or she to know their father and other members of their paternal family, especially if you have grown up without a father or paternal relatives yourself.

Abandoned Pregnant

It is not good to deprive children of getting to know their father, but you love them so much you want to protect them from getting hurt.

There are ways you can try to make things work, such as meeting with your child's father for the first time alone, without your child being there.

Speak with him in a neutral location, like a park or a public coffee house, and converse with him at great length about his intentions. Make it clear that you will not accept him coming in and out of your child's life, he has to be sure that this is what he wants, as you will not put your child through this, only to be let down by his/her father.

When you meet with your ex, it is important that you have no expectations such as gifts or money for your child or even an apology for that matter.

Of course he *should* apologise and show some sort of remorse for how he treated you during your pregnancy, but if he doesn't, don't say anything to him about it, as you are not there to receive an apology or to speak about the past which will definitely stir old feelings and things will quickly turn nasty; you are there to speak about your child getting to know his or her father. The fact that he doesn't apologise or mention anything about what happened during your pregnancy might not mean that he isn't sorry or that he doesn't care; he might be embarrassed and not know what to say to you just yet. Give it some time, he might just surprise you by his actions and efforts into being a father.

Abandoned Pregnant

At first you will understandably not want to send your child with their father alone on visits, so you will both have to come to an arrangement about how he will have contact with his child, until you are comfortable enough with being able to let your child go with their father by himself or herself.
You could start off at neutral meeting places, then, when you are ready to make progress, you could go to wherever he lives, so that you can see where he will be taking your child before sending them off with him somewhere you don't know it's safe etc.
A lot of trust has been lost throughout what happened during your pregnancy, the time when you needed him most; he should expect not be in for an easy ride. Your ex now has to prove himself.

If for some reason things don't go well – for example, your ex repeatedly not showing up for contact with his child on schedules days without informing you that he won't be able to come, or if he is taking more of an interest in trying to get back with you than paying any attention to his child – then you might want to consider not having him around.
Your ex needs to genuinely want to be a father to his child and his actions will tell you just that: remember, don't ignore any signs.
If your ex has a partner and you don't feel comfortable with sending your child around to his place, then that could create a problem.

Abandoned Pregnant

As hard as it is to accept this would happen someday, your ex was not going to remain single forever. If you have moved on and also have a partner who spends time around your child, then there shouldn't be an issue with your ex's partner being able to do the same. Your ex should have quality time with your child sometimes, when it is just the two of them; his partner should not be involved in every contact. If this seems to become an issue, then politely tell him that you are sure your child would like some time with just daddy.
Hopefully he should get the message.
If your ex happens to live with his partner, then your child is bound to form some sort of relationship with her, but the same statement applies that there should be times when he has days out or does an activity with his dad alone, just one on one time.

If a situation arises where your ex becomes disrespectful to you, shout at you, or call you names, you do not have to tolerate it, not even for your child.
If you find that he is a good father to your child, but there seems to be an issue whenever he sees you, then it would be best to try another alternative than having to see him.
If you have a mutual friend or anybody that could be present for these contact or whenever your child is being collected and dropped back home, then that should avoid any communication or confrontation between the two of you.

But how long can that last? Can you really have someone present all the time when it comes to dealing with you ex? Nobody was present when you both created your child, so you both at some point need to work out a way to come to some mutual understanding about what is best for your child. That is not to see the parents arguing every time daddy comes over or when it's time to go to daddy's house or come back home to mummy.
It's unsettling for the child, especially at such a young age.

If your ex makes contact with you about wanting to now be a father to his child and you know he is not going to do anything good in your child's life, but will become a potential bad influence, if you think that your child could possibly become a victim of their fathers bad or violent behaviour and only end up hurt, then make the right choice and protect your child.
Other downfalls in the father of your child, you need to leave down to your child to find out first hand. He or she can decide as to whether or not they really want a relationship with him later.
Remember that children don't stay children; they grow up. You don't want your child resenting you over not knowing their father because you didn't allow it over a reason that doesn't make sense to them.
When you see your ex, old feelings might come flooding back, but think back to the way he treated you when

you were pregnant with his child. He should look a lot uglier after that.

If he flirts with you, mentions he is singe or wants to try to become a family and that's what you want too, you need to be so very careful about this because it is too soon and things will end in disaster. Rushing into anything without discussing what happened between you both during your pregnancy, overlooking that, would be sweeping the mess under the carpet until someone moves the rug.

To have a successful relationship with this man, you will both need to go to couples counselling and deal with everything. If not, don't be surprised when, less than six months into the relationship, during an argument, you find yourself hurling the past in his face about how he left you while you were carrying his baby.

I don't recommend going back to your ex at all: this man ditched you at a time in your life when you were most vulnerable, he let you down then, when you needed him most, and he will more than likely let you down again. Could you really trust him again after everything that's happened? Don't get caught up on the idea of becoming a family, the thought of your child being raised by their mum and dad is a lovely one, but not if your child is unhappy because mum and dad are unhappy too.

The father of my first child and I did that, I know we loved each other very much, but I think we both, deep down, got back together for our daughter's sake, to try to be a family.

Abandoned Pregnant

When I left the relationship I was in to get back with him, the main reason was because he was my daughter's dad and I wanted her to grow up living with a mummy and a daddy. It was the same reason that kept us from breaking up when our relationship had broken down: our daughter. Our relationship had got so bad, to the point where we would tell each other so. We failed to realise what we were doing not only to ourselves, but to our daughter too.

Chapter 18
Reconciling with your ex

I know, I know... Some of you are thinking "no way would I ever get back with that loser," but it does happen. It happened to me, never say never.
You might not even see it coming - I certainly didn't, my ex and I pretty much got back together the very first day we saw each other again after he left me pregnant.
Again, I know... Sounds crazy, right? I was so happy to be with the father of my child again, I didn't think twice, I got out of the relationship I was in at once, without a thought for how my boyfriend at the time felt. Honestly, I didn't care either, I was in my own element, my little cloud of happiness.
That's where I went wrong, I rushed back into a relationship with my ex and I didn't observe him to see if he had changed or make him work to earn my trust and respect after what he had put me through.
I should have suggested we went to counselling to see if we could make the relationship work after everything we had been through. I made everything too easy for him and that is because I didn't love or respect myself enough then.
If you find yourself in a situation where you and your ex still have strong feelings for each other and you want to try to make things work properly, it is going to take time, don't immediately go back to how things were like I did with my ex.

Abandoned Pregnant

We briefly discussed what had happened between us, but it was very short; he did say he was sorry, he did tell me he had missed me and had thought about me, amongst other things that made me happy to hear.
That was nine years ago and back then, that was enough for me... It was good enough for me and I accepted it. I didn't realise I was, in fact, showing him that it was ok to do something seriously wrong, that I would take him back with an apology and the nice things he said, that I would even leave a relationship I was in for him. He knew at that point that he could basically come in and out of my life when he wanted.
He knew I put him on a pedestal simply because he was the father of my child. Which is why, when we had our problems, he would tell me that we were not together anymore one day, then the next day he would say we were. I had given him that power to control our relationship and tell me when we were together and when we were not.
Please do not get caught up in that trap like I did, it took him leaving me again for me to learn my lesson.

Do not take your ex back as quickly as I did, this is something that should take a few months to work on and it would benefit you both massively if you went for counselling together to discuss past issues and his absence during your pregnancy.
It is important that you are both honest in counselling or it will not work. From there, you will know if you can figure out a way forward into a reconciliation.

Abandoned Pregnant

Do not become intimate in any way with your ex until you have moved past your issues, as it will only complicate your emotions and make things worse.
Your ex will need to earn your trust again and prove to you that he is capable of being a good father to his child and a good partner to you. Things are not the same as when you were last together, there is another person to consider now, your child.
Do not allow your ex to move in right away either, take things very slowly. This man has caused you a lot of hurt and pain, the fact that you are even considering getting back into a relationship with him again is really something...
Don't tell a lot of people about your plans to reconcile with your ex, as their responses may leave you feeling stupid; they will not understand why you would want to do such a thing, isn't this the same man that said he didn't want his own child and left you to manage alone? Didn't this man have you in a state close to emotional wreck? But time has a way of making us forget the bad times and remember the good ones.
 People who care about you would be well within their rights to have concerns or even be angry with you, it's only because they don't want to see you hurt again.
There are some women who would view negative responses from their friends as them being jealous, but I very much doubt that they are; they are just trying to make you see things from the outside point of view. Imagine if a friend of yours had been through what you had, only to announce that they planned to get back

with the man who put her through such an awful ordeal... What would you say to her? What would you think about her? Would you lose respect for her?

Your family are, no doubt, bound not to be impressed by your decision either, but hopefully you will still have their support, should you need it.

You need to be sure that getting back together with your ex is what you really want and consider if it is in the best interests of your child.

Make sure you are not considering getting back with your ex just because you are lonely and have no man in your life. If you reconcile with your ex simply because of that reason, including the fact he is the father of your baby, then you will never move on. Your ex will get in the way of you ever meeting a new potential partner and you will end up with a life that you are unhappy with.

Respecting yourself and loving yourself enough will prevent you from making this mistake; the same goes for the situation when your ex only wants to be intimate with you, but doesn't want a relationship.

Do not allow him to use you like that after the way he has disrespected you!

Do not allow yourself to be mistreated, hoping that sleeping with him will eventually turn into a relationship, because it won't! You will be giving him everything he wants for nothing; he's not your boyfriend, so you can't have any expectations. He can do whatever he wants and would not want to ruin that by committing himself to you after you have already given him all of you. Don't put yourself back into a crisis, you know what this man is capable of; you can forgive but do not forget, because that would be stupid, you need to learn from the lesson to make sure it doesn't happen again. Do not allow an immature and irresponsible man to destroy your life.

Again, if you love and respect yourself, you should be strong enough to prevent this from happening to you. If it does happen, you need to start learning self-love and self-worth.

Sometimes people change and have a good reconciliation, but most never end that way and the divide only becomes bigger.

If you have come a long way and your ex now wants to reconcile, but you are not too sure about it then don't do it; please do not regress all the positive work you have done, stay strong and wait for Mr Right.

A love that is strong will leave you with feelings that last after a relationship ends; love can still exist long after terrible things have been done to you, even though your heart got broken, but just because you might still be in love with your ex doesn't mean that you should be with him, especially if the relationship is no longer healthy.

Chapter 19
Be Grateful For What You Do Have

We are all guilty of taking the good things in our lives for granted, and we are all guilty of always wanting to have more. While it is important to strive in life, it is also very important at times that we stop to appreciate what we have and what we have already accomplished, or else you may end up feeling like a puppy running around and around trying to catch its tail.
Focus on what you have, not on what is missing.
Appreciating all the things you have in your life can empower you, because you can focus on all the things you have done to be able to get as far as you have in your life. Appreciate and be proud of what you have earned for yourself already and believe in your ability to achieve the next level until you get what you really want.
It will not be easy, but by moving through this chapter in your life, you will learn to appreciate and be grateful for what you do have with or without the father of your child.
Being left to raise a baby alone proves that you are not always in control of your own life, life is just going to keep happening to you without your consent. What you have let to learn, life will always find a way to teach you, but things will be ok.

Abandoned Pregnant

You are human, you have the ability to grow and to change. With self-reflection and a positive, healthy attitude towards your future, you will indeed be ok.

Don't close yourself off, be open to meeting new people and be open to falling in love again. Love can only blossom if you are open to love in your life, set that intention for love to enter your life.

I know that feeling when you say to yourself 'if I keep people at arm's length, then they can't hurt me.' While you will avoid being hurt by others by closing yourself off from them, the downside is that you will also be missing out on happiness. Be yourself: you will attract people who are suited for you.

Be yourself, instead of hiding behind a mask pretending to be someone you are not.

Try to let go and stop repeating the story of what happened between you and the father of your child to yourself; it could be blocking you from having love enter your life again, carrying that sort of energy around with you.

It's only after you have lost everything that you are free to see what you were missing out on; being single, you now have an opportunity to do all the things you put off while you were busy fixating all your energy into trying to make things with your ex work out. I believe that being single is a call to focus on yourself. Sometimes, being in a relationship can make you too comfortable; you become lazy about developing yourself and any goals you once had end up taking a back seat.

Abandoned Pregnant

Don't ever feel that your life is over, you are only just beginning your new life as a mother and have plenty to look forward to; it might not seem like it now, but you do.

You are alive, you are healthy and you are going to experience the most amazing thing that a woman can ever do, give life. Be grateful you have been blessed to know this feeling as not all women can in their lives.

Be thankful that your pregnancy is progressing and your baby is healthy and safe.

Chapter 20
Dealing With Depression

It can be an emotional time, coping with heartbreak on top of all the hormonal activity going on, triggering mood swings. There isn't much support for pregnant single women being heartbroken during pregnancy, which is sad, considering how many women are going through it; it's like our feelings aren't being accounted for and it's our fault for being in this predicament.

Women are expected to look good and feel great during their 'blooming' nine months - thanks to pregnant celebrities and models - but the reality is very different for a woman who is suffering with depression during her pregnancy.

Just like postnatal depression, antenatal depression can strike at any moment in pregnancy.

Even if you were depressed at the beginning of your pregnancy, you could find that during your last trimester, bitter feelings towards your child's father and your situation intensify.

Such feelings can lead to sadness and confusion, maybe even concerns about not being ready to become a mum, or fears about the birth.

Depression and anxiety often goes on undiagnosed, because women dismiss their feelings and put them down to temporary moodiness that accompanies pregnancy.

Abandoned Pregnant

Let your midwife know if you are feeling low, it is important because depression does not only affect your health, but can also harm your unborn baby; so do not be afraid to get help.
Some symptoms of depression include feelings of helplessness and hopelessness, changes in your sleeping pattern, weight changes, reckless behaviour, anger, etc.

There are ways you can try to manage and relieve the symptoms of depression, like yoga, which helps to calm the mind and alleviate aches and pains.
Try to stay connected with friends and family, don't stay in bed all day, isolating yourself will make your symptoms worse.
Getting enough sleep when you are pregnant is hard enough, let alone trying to sleep for eight hours, but getting eight hours of sleep can help improve your mood.
Find support; whether it be an online support group forum or a group support session talking to other women who can relate to what you are going through; it can make a difference.
Getting professional help, like a counsellor is definitely something you need to do if everything is becoming too much for you and you feel overwhelmed with a lack of support around you. Letting things out is good for us, there are things we will tell counsellor that we would not tell our friends, and that includes our honesty about how we really feel, because we know what we are

saying is in complete confidentiality. We don't have to lie or pretend.

If you are worried about income or finances, there are a number of services the government provides to help with food, clothing, housing, day-care etc. Call your local job centre to find out any benefits you may be entitled to, and visit your local council to see how they might be able to also help you with council tax, rent, etc.

Depression that is left untreated can be very dangerous, for both mother and baby, so please do not ignore any signs or symptoms that suggest you might be suffering with the illness.

At the beginning of this book, I told you about the time I was on the floor, eight months pregnant, crying. I was depressed then and went to my doctor to be referred for counselling.

I will never forget how alone I felt and how angry I was that nobody around me seemed to truly understand the pain I was in or how much what my ex had done had affected me.

I felt like I wanted to scream and punch something.

The anxiety I suffered during my second pregnancy, hoping and waiting for my ex to come back to me, was awful I was behaving recklessly by sending blackberry broadcasts around to my contacts about him. I remember when people would congratulate me and assume how happy I must be, but I wasn't, not really, and I felt guilty for not being happy. I was unhappy with

Abandoned Pregnant

my situation, not being pregnant, and I didn't get to enjoy most of my pregnancy because of that.

Don't allow that to happen to you, take control if you are depressed and seek help among doing things to help relieve symptoms of depression. Medication, like anti-depressants, can be prescribed by your doctor, however treatment will depend on the severity of your depression; your doctor may just recommend and refer you to a counsellor or a therapist.

It is important you address and get help with serious issues of depression before your baby arrives, otherwise you may struggle in taking care of you both and everything might feel as if it's becoming too much to cope with.

Make sure you don't sit in silence if you are depressed, let your nearest and dearest be aware of how you feel, so they too can become more involved in supporting you through this difficult time.

Please remember that you are not worthless, you are a woman who is about to do the most rewarding job on earth, become a mum and your baby is going to need you and love you very much.

If you are experiencing dangerous or suicidal thoughts then please call the Samaritans or someone close to you for help.

Your situation is not permanent, but ending your life is.

Chapter 21
You will survive

It took me just under five years to get over my second ex who left me pregnant. I remember a time when I was in tears, thinking there was something wrong with me, because I couldn't stop thinking about him and just move on. I had several years' worth of memories with him and it took me half the time I had known him to fully get over him.
I no longer miss him anymore, he isn't a part of my daily thoughts or conversations, and in fact if I am honest I'm not even attracted to him anymore!
I've seen pictures of him on mutual friends' Facebook timelines and I feel nothing. I think "oh wow, I wouldn't even look at this type of man now." My taste in men has totally change, because I am now more in touch with myself, I have taken the time to get to understand my personality, and I know who I am and what I want.
I want you to also take this time being single to get to know yourself and what it is that you want, it doesn't even need to be about a relationship; it could be about a plan, a goal, or something else.
Being in a relationship is not important, especially now. What is important is your baby and as long as you are doing what you are supposed to as a mother, then everything will be ok, things will fall into place; slowly but surely.

Abandoned Pregnant

Don't spend time worrying or wondering about how you are going to cope, realise that you are in fact already coping and have coped through the situation this far. The time you spend feeling frustrated that you cannot seem to get over your ex is actually all a part of the process of you moving on; you just don't realise it.

Stick to whatever you are doing that helps you to express your feelings whether that's counselling, writing down your feelings, exercise etc. Keeping busy will definitely help you to stay focused on what you are doing.

Your thinking changes after you have a baby: you mature, you don't have time for what you once did and wonder why you even made time for some of the things you used to do as they might seem silly to you now. The same goes for people that you know: some of the people you once were close with, you find you now have nothing in common with since having your baby if any of your friends aren't parents themselves; or maybe you don't want their lifestyles around your baby.

You may even not stay in contact with some of them anymore, since your lifestyle has changed and you have now become a mother.

This isn't a bad thing: you know what you want and what you don't want in your child's life. The fact that you are making your life a safe zone for your baby is great! Protect them from any possible bad influences early in their lives, as children can still pick up learnt behaviour from other people who they see often.

Abandoned Pregnant

If you have been avoiding Rom-Coms like I did when I was pregnant, it's actually not a bad idea to watch some now, but in moderation like once a month. People tend to think that by not watching romantic films or comedies, they won't have to feel sad or get emotional. But the real reason they avoid these shows is because they have not dealt with their own issues in their break up and are still holding onto feelings. Watching romance is not a bad thing as it puts the idea of possibly ever finding love back into your mind.

I am single, and right now I have no problem in watching a RomCom on my own; I will even laugh if it's funny. Five years ago I could have never done that, but since putting some serious work into myself, I've realised that I am able to do anything I choose to put my mind to - within reason - and so can you.

You've got to tell yourself that you will survive, and you've got to believe it.

Every day that goes, by milestones will be reached, while your old world ended with 'lasts' your new world is full of 'firsts.'

The first time you don't think about him, not even once, from the moment you woke up until the moment it was bedtime again.

The first time you realise you didn't cry today.

The first time you laugh so hard, you can't remember when last you actually laughed like that.

The first time you really understand what "moving on" truly means.

Abandoned Pregnant

The first time it hits you, you've survived being left pregnant.

Abandoned Pregnant

Now You're Ready, Get Your Pen Out!

Write out a list, make notes of the positives and the negatives about your situation as a single mum.

Abandoned Pregnant

Abandoned Pregnant

Abandoned Pregnant

This section is for the negative stuff you listed; work out if you can turn them into positives and how to go about it.

Abandoned Pregnant

Abandoned Pregnant

Abandoned Pregnant

Write a plan of action for the negatives
that can be changed into positives.

Abandoned Pregnant

Abandoned Pregnant

Abandoned Pregnant

Now put your plan into action!
Start another list; this time you will be writing about your friendships and relationships with the people in your life, do you still want some of these people around now you are a mum? Be honest with yourself and decide to let go if those who are not good for you and won't set positive examples for your child.

Make notes of all the things you are looking forward to doing with and for your baby. Jot down the advantages and benefits of being a single mum.

Abandoned Pregnant

Abandoned Pregnant

Abandoned Pregnant

Write down how it feels trying to get your ex to be a father; vent out your frustrations, his responses to what you have said to him about the situation, and your result at the end.

Abandoned Pregnant

Abandoned Pregnant

Make a list of all the things you think you need from your ex during your pregnancy and in the beginning stages of your child's life, you may find you will struggle to get past number 2.

Abandoned Pregnant

Abandoned Pregnant

Abandoned Pregnant

Make a list of all your qualities you know that have value, then write a brief essay about all of those qualities and values, one at a time. Read what you have written whenever you feel low.

Abandoned Pregnant

Abandoned Pregnant

Abandoned Pregnant

Save everything you have written as when you one day in the future you will see how far you have come.

Look back at what you have written whenever you feel the urge to speak with your ex about being a father again, to remind yourself why you should stay away from him.

Abandoned Pregnant

Remember To...

Keep a journal you can write in daily about your thoughts and feelings to let off steam.

Think positive.

Divert any thoughts about your ex into something out of your comfort zone, whether it be a new interest, hobbies, new book, etc.

Speak with a counsellor to be able to release negative feelings about your ex and the situation he has left you in.

Join antenatal classes, support groups for single parents etc.

Don't pay gossips any attention, think about whether what these people think really matters.

It's good to talk sometimes, but be careful about whom you confide in, and about the company you keep around you.

Abandoned Pregnant

Do not allow yourself to become influenced by bad examples, no matter who they are being set by. They make things worse for you and it's you who has to suffer any consequences alone.

Think about how you will inform family members about your pregnancy and your relationship breakdown.

Remember all the reasons why you decided to keep your baby

STOP waiting for your ex to come back. Look over all you have written down and see if your ex's behaviours are the actions of a man who wants to be with you and have a baby.

BELIEVE you CAN raise your child on your own without his or her father. You don't need him!

Don't have any expectations of your ex.

LOVE YOURSELF

Think of others who are less fortunate and other women who have been in this situation before you, remember you are not alone in this.

Try to be around positivity.

Abandoned Pregnant

Start learning from your experience.

Stop living in denial.

Think about who you were before you met your ex and how you can get your mind back to the way it used to before he was constantly on it. You could get back to that state of mind - only better, now you have had this experience to teach you lesson, and gained wisdom.

Remember that not everyone who comes into your life will have a purpose to stay in it.

THINK before you react! Take time to let the news about your ex moving on sink in.

Remember that whoever your ex chooses to see is none of your business.

Learn to allow your ex to live with the choices he makes without getting involved, trying to show him the error of his ways.

Learn to live with the choices you have made in your situation.

Don't forget the way your ex has treated you; if he could this to you, he could do it to another woman too.

Abandoned Pregnant

Do not allow the situation to take over your thoughts - keep busy!

Avoid attempting to make contact with your ex's new girlfriend, for your own feelings sake.

Consider the fact that even if your ex did want to be in your child's life, but not in a relationship with you, you would have to accept the fact that he would meet someone else at some point - and at some stage, your ex's new partner would probably become involved in your child's life.

Don't waste time trying to defend yourself about the paternity of your child, if your ex is telling people that he is not the father. They don't really care and you will only be drawing more attention to your situation.

Even if your ex denies his paternity, if you need financial help from him once your baby is born, you can still apply to the child support maintenance service and leave it to them to sort it out. As I stated earlier they will organise a DNA test for you all, and if your ex fails to attend, then his parentage is assumed and deductions will be made from his income.

Your ex will not feel sorry for you by you pestering him about the situation every day.

Abandoned Pregnant

Show your ex that you are moving forward with your life by not contacting him. He has made his choice so any communication now has to come from him.

Think: if your ex was around, would it be in the best interest of your child?

Let go of any hope you may have been holding onto that your ex would return.

Give yourself advice that you would give a friend or family member in your situation.

Don't keep track of when you last saw your ex, it only hurts you every time you're aware another day has passed by.

Be honest with your family about what is happening so you can receive the support you need.

Try to remember that all the confusion and mixed emotions you are experiencing are normal for a woman in your circumstance.

Remember that you cannot compare your situation to anyone else's, as everybody is different.

Stop going over everything trying to make sense of it all as it only leads to more confusion.

Abandoned Pregnant

Don't stalk your ex's social network pages - you won't be doing yourself any favours!

Make the decision of whether you are going to cut off your ex completely, or just have no contact until he chooses otherwise.

You will feel happier not wasting energy trying to change things that you cannot.

Remember, things will become easier as you adapt; it won't always be like this.

Make a decision so you are not waiting in hope: are you going to allow your ex contact in the future if he wants, or is he totally out if the picture?

Think about the things you can change.

A wake up call is not a bad thing. It can create opportunities to make corrections in your life

Be consistent in making the changes you need to improve your life.

Any goal you want to achieve, write it down and work towards it every day.

Believe in yourself.

Abandoned Pregnant

Say positive things about yourself and your goals out loud; saying things out loud makes them become real.

Do things that make you happy

Don't contact your ex after you have had your baby, he will know your due date (I'm sure you told him!) trying to get him to take notice of you and your baby will only cause you more disappointment.

Do not send your ex photos of your baby.
If he would like to see the baby I'm sure he knows where you live, or he can contact you somehow.

Do not call or text your ex about your baby.

Remember, it's your ex's loss and not yours.

If your ex wants back in, and you want to try again too, don't allow him to re-enter your lives too easily - make him earn your trust.

Avoid stressful situations.

Think about other positive male role models you might have in your life, who could be good father figures for your child, and don't reunite with your ex for the sake of being a family.

Do not allow what your ex has done to you make you have false beliefs about yourself.

Do not blame yourself, as you only feed the rejection by doing that.

Don't forget that what you are feeling now is temporary.

Rejection can happen to anyone

Don't suppress your feelings, express them through conversations with someone you can trust whether that's family or friends or a new hobby like art.

Do not distance yourself from others as you will feel even more alone and as if nobody cares about you.

Let go of your mistakes. Mistakes happen to everyone. Take what you can from them, learn from them, and then move on.

Embrace your future.

Abandoned Pregnant

Celebrate your past, it might be hard for you, but without your past, you wouldn't be where you are today.

Sing your own praises once in a while

Remember that having love and respect for yourself gives you a better life.

Be patient with yourself, the change won't take place over night.

Stop any self-criticism.

Listen to your gut feeling.

Remember that your child will be learning and being taught about self-love and respect from what you are displaying.

Do not get into another relationship unless you are ready to do so, and it is what you want.

Choose the things that really matter.

Choose the right perspective.

Break away from old habits.

Abandoned Pregnant

Change your lifestyle.

Remember to get rid of an old bedding you once shared with your ex.

Dive into new hobbies or old passions.

Tell your child about their father in simple terms they can understand, don't make it confusing for them.

Make sure your child knows that they are loved and they are not to blame.

Avoid lying to your child.

Allow your child to express how they feel.

Do not speak badly about your ex in front of your child.

Take notice of any after-reactions.

If your ex happens to want to re-enter your life make him earn the right and your trust before you even consider reconciling.

Before getting into any relationship make sure it is want, don't allow yourself to be pushed into anything unless you are ready for it.

Abandoned Pregnant

Keep both eyes and ears open for any signs that start to show your partners true colours.

Read good books on new relationships.

Always put your child's needs before any man's, including their father's.

Do not have your new partner around your child 247; take the introduction process slowly.

Get to know your partner properly, meet his family and friends.

Figure out what you want in your life and what you don't want.

Seeking revenge is only going to make the situation worse, not better.

You may end up unintentionally hurting other people who are innocent in the process of trying to get back at your ex.

Replace negative feelings of revenge with positive thinking.

Leave any ill feelings of revenge for the universe to handle, karma is a bitch.

Abandoned Pregnant

Don't forget, living well is the best revenge.

Seeking revenge will change others opinions about you; if they felt sorry for you before they won't after you carry out your plans and you could end up turning people against you.

Try to make peace with yourself instead of making plans for revenge.

Spend your time doing something constructive, rather than pranking your ex like I did; it didn't change anything and was a waste of my time.

Golden rule - refrain from speaking negatively about your ex to his family members - especially his mum!

Avoid entering into any form of discussion regarding your relationship with your ex in front of his family members.

Do not lose focus of what is supposed to be happening, any interaction you have with your ex's mother, or other family members, is meant to be for contact between them and your child, not an opportunity to speak about your ex.

Don't take out stored up, negative feelings over your ex on his family.

Abandoned Pregnant

Set the standard of how you are treated from the beginning.

Never get too comfortable with your ex's relatives; don't forget, these people are your child's family, not yours.

When meeting with your child's father for the first time since you have had your baby, do not expect anything such as money or gifts for your child - or an apology for the way he has treated you.

Decide on meeting locations that are neutral.

Never say never, as anything can happen.

Don't rush back into a relationship with your ex.

Make your ex earn your trust again.

Remember that it is a slow process.

Persuade your ex to go to counselling with you as one of the mandatory things that needs to happen before you can get back together if that is what you want.

Remember that negative comments made by friends and family are to be expected, as they are only looking out for you.

Abandoned Pregnant

Imagine a friend was in your situation, what would you say to her?

Do not forget what your ex has put you through and how it made you feel; can you really move past everything with him?

Remember: you need to do what is in the best interests of your child. You don't want them growing up in a war zone.

If you are unsure that you want to get back into a relationship with your ex and need to think about it, then don't go back. If you really wanted to be with him you would know straight away.

Abandoned Pregnant

Dear Reader, I wish you all the best during your amazing journey through pregnancy, and I hope that you have a safe delivery, as well as a healthy baby.
Stay Strong.
Kandy

Abandoned Pregnant

About The Author

Kandy Dolor was born in 1985 and lives in London.

Kandy Dolor is the Author of KandyCares Self Help Books which she writes with qualifications of experience from her own life experiences.
The purpose of KandyCares Self Help Books is to help women who may be going through hard times in life that the author can relate to.
Kandy Dolor is available to give talks at centres, group meetings, conferences, functions and all other events.
You can enquire using the contact details below.
You can also get in touch if you are interested in the author covering a subject you would like to read more about.
www.kandycares.org
kandycaresbooks@gmail.com
https://www.facebook.com/KandyCaresSelfHelpBooks

Abandoned Pregnant

Abandoned Pregnant

My Notes

Abandoned Pregnant

My Notes

Abandoned Pregnant

Abandoned Pregnant

Abandoned Pregnant

Printed in Great Britain
by Amazon